Praise for Sisterhood in Sports

"A detailed, enlightening look at a fascinating topic that all coaches of women and girls should be highly interested in."

—**Mike Woitalla**, *executive editor,* Soccer America

"Sisterhood in Sports *provides a unique view of the challenges, emotional highs and lows, and importance of connected relationships for female athletes. As an athlete and sport psychologist who has lived through the evolution of the modern female athlete, Dr. Joan Steidinger provides an engaging look of the roles of friends, family, teammates, coaches, parents, motherhood, and romantic relationships that are unique for female athletes at varying stages of life. As an athlete and a mother, I'm excited to see a rare, but needed, book full of female athlete stories."*

—**Danelle Kabush**, *PhD, professional off-road triathlete, LUNA pro team; Xterra triathlon; mental performance consultant; mother*

"I had Dr. Joan Steidinger come and talk and work with my women's track and cross country teams, and the results were unbelievable. Through Steidinger's instruction and guidance she taught them how to tap into their true potential. I believe the wisdom and suggestions Dr. Joan Steidinger shares in this book, Sisterhood in Sports, *can help others achieve their true potential."*

—**Ken Grace**, *head track coach, Chabot College; health/kinesiology instructor; CoachCalifornia community coach of the year*

"I wish that I could have read Sisterhood in Sports *thirty years ago. Now, thanks to Dr. Joan Steidinger, I am empowered to encourage collaborative competition, embrace my strength, and teach others how to do the same."*

—**Shana Bagley**, *esq., Clipper Cup racer; double-handed ocean racer; Ragnar and Tough Mudder runner; strongman, Highland Games; men's rugby national finalist*

SISTERHOOD IN SPORTS

SISTERHOOD IN SPORTS

How Female Athletes Collaborate and Compete

Joan Steidinger

ROWMAN & LITTLEFIELD
Lanham • Boulder • New York • London

Published by Rowman & Littlefield
A wholly owned subsidiary of The Rowman & Littlefield Publishing Group, Inc.
4501 Forbes Boulevard, Suite 200, Lanham, Maryland 20706
www.rowman.com

16 Carlisle Street, London W1D 3BT, United Kingdom

British Library Cataloguing in Publication Information Available

Library of Congress Cataloging-in-Publication Data

Steidinger, Joan.
Sisterhood in sports : how female athletes collaborate and compete / Joan Steidinger.
pages cm
Includes bibliographical references and index.
ISBN 978-1-4422-3033-0 (cloth : alk. paper) -- ISBN 978-1-4422-3034-7 (electronic)
1. Sports for women. 2. Women athletes. 3. Women athletes--Psychology. I. Title.
GV709.S74 2014
796.082--dc23
2014016818

Printed in the United States of America

To my mother, Frances Palmer Steidinger, the athlete who taught me loving kindness and provided support when it was important, whom I "speak out" for now.

CONTENTS

AUTHOR'S NOTES

Twenty years in the unfolding, *Sisterhood in Sports* made for an amazing journey. My sports interest and involvement have stretched throughout the course of my lifetime. The lesson I took from running in my first marathon in 1987 was the wonderful camaraderie of training in groups and learning to feel more comfortable about my body. Although running with both women and men, I talked to my girlfriends about relationships. The first germs of wanting to write a book about female athletes started as I began making notes and writing down ideas in 1994, shortly after completing the Western States one-hundred-mile race. During that time, my eye was often on Ann Trason. Ann's toughness and ability to beat almost everyone (she came in second in Western States 100 in 1994 and 1995) led the way for women in the ultra world. The idea continued after I watched the 1996 US Olympic women's soccer team win gold at the Olympics. The tight bond evident among the "Fab Five" of soccer, Kristine Lilly (interviewed for this book), Julie Foudy, Brandi Chastain, Joy Fawcett, and Mia Hamm—a bond that persists to this day—was inspirational. Whenever the Olympics come around, the television is constantly on.

In 1997, as I was emerging from a difficult relationship that derailed my training and competitiveness as an ultrarunner, my curiosity peaked about female athletes, relationships, and competitive sports. As a way to mend, I trained and rode my first double century, where I met my husband, JP. I would be remiss if I didn't mention how much the support of my husband has meant to me. He arrived in my life six months after my breakup, initially noticing me at the end of the double century bike ride. He's always said, "I like those big strong girl athletes." He has watched me agonize over this project over the past seventeen years, providing support and love.

As a lifelong athlete raised by a mother and father who were athletes, I actually began my journey by looking back at the family members and a coach who impacted me over the years. As I was growing up, each of my parents shared a gift with me: kindness and thoughtfulness from my southern English mother and mental toughness from my German Irish father. In contrast to my competitive father, my mother, Frances, was a shy and make-nice kind of person; 5'8" and athletic, she played a strong game of golf; but my father, Dean, was so tough on my mom that it seemed to hurt her game. My father was a talented golfer himself, with a 6/7 handicap; they both loved the game. Inheriting his tenacity (he played golf for over seventy-five years) has served me well my whole life in all my pursuits. Moving around to different states, the family always managed to end up attached to golf and country clubs with swimming pools. Playing golf and swimming began at a very young age for me. My parents exposed their only child to a whole bunch of other sports, including horseback riding, canoeing, hiking, backpacking, synchronized swimming, badminton, tennis, bike riding, and much more. Despite only sporadically attending my sports competitions, my parents were both athletic role models to me.

The one coach who stands out for me is Ken Grace. He helped me more than even he knows. By introducing me to the heart rate monitor, he empowered me to push myself to limits I did not know I could achieve. His positive and upbeat attitude whenever we spoke helped my confidence grow, which laid the groundwork for my running my first one-hundred-mile race in 1992 (Vermont), finishing in under twenty-four hours, beating five horses (concurrent horse endurance race), and placing tenth woman. Eventually, the following season, my team won first place in the Pacific Region Ultra Series, and I managed to finish third in the Open Division of that same series.

When I began this project seriously in 1997 by writing my first proposal, my focus was on interviewing forty female ultrarunners about how their interpersonal relationships impacted their ultrarunning and sporting life. The ultrarunning community had created a home of sorts. Martha Cederstrom, a former ultrarunner, has remained a constant friend. We're still running buddies, and the friendship remains strong to this day. Submission of the first proposal taught me about rejection early in the process, although I did interview over forty female ultrarunners afterward in 1998. I've learned over the years that rejection of a book proposal is merely a business decision and not personal.

In the following years, my work focused on providing sports psychology services, teaching classes on the subject at UC Berkeley Extension, and serving as a guest speaker at venues throughout California. My passion for sports psychology grew each time I spoke about it. All this became a way for me to build further expertise and gain credibility and further experience for writing the book.

Then in September of 2003—just as my practice in sports psychology was taking off—I was involved in a serious bicycle accident. This landed me in the hospital with multiple injuries for a couple of weeks. I couldn't walk on my own due to six pelvic fractures until December of that year, slept on a wedge pillow for six months, and did not have a completely clear mind due to the seriousness of the concussion received. The accident also caused three broken ribs and required rotator cuff rebuild surgery.

Slowly rehabbing in the months that followed, I never returned to my previous form. Prior to the accident, I had participated in long-distance competitive trail running (ultrarunning) and done reasonably well, and I was riding double centuries regularly with my husband. JP and I rode the triple crown one year (three double centuries in one year). In 2003, before the mishap, I had finished second Masters in the worst weather conditions of the Catalina Trail Marathon in the twenty-six-year history of the race and rode Davis Double Century shortly afterward. My initial limited mobility, along with a subsequent cancer diagnosis for my husband, diverted my attention from my athletic pursuits. There were other priorities. My attention was completely focused on JP and his survival. This was a painful time for both of us, but we both persevered and survived.

Many months later, I was unable to run and found it difficult to climb mountains on bicycles without significant pelvic pain. The following year, I attempted the Death Ride but only managed four passes with my injuries. Climbing continual uphills is hard on someone who's had multiple pelvis fractures, which can be painful and frustrating when you were previously a strong climber. Needing to turn my attention away from sports for a while, I established a Vietnamese embroidered silk jacket import business for several years—it was successful but not my real passion. I was fifty years old, and this was my midlife crisis. After I had traveled back and forth to Vietnam over ten times, my interest returned to sports, and I hoped to return to running, albeit it slowly.

Finally, in 2009, the book idea emerged again, and my focus was back on sports psychology. My first step was to join a writer's salon, Left Coast Writers, and a writer's club, California Writer's Club–Marin. Thanks to my friend Patti (Katz) Chang, my first interview was with Olympic cyclist and physician Christine Thorburn, whom she knew. Patti, who's a University of California, San Francisco, researcher and tenured professor, encouraged me to refocus on the book. In addition, as I had rejoined the Association of Applied Sports Psychology, the direct networking began again. The interviews continued through 2010 and 2011 with Olympians, professionals, elite amateurs, and recreational female athletes. At the same time, another proposal emerged with the help of Jordan Rosenfeld. I pitched it for six months with different publishers and agents. Despite having the proposal read a number of times, I faced the rejection parade again.

Not to be deterred, I made it my mission to find another book coach for a fresh perspective (Brooke Warner), establish better organization, and do another rewrite. As I wrote, I continued to build my expertise. In late summer 2011, I applied and, after a rigorous process, was accepted as a certified consultant by the Association of Applied Sports Psychology. In November 2012, I was placed on the US Olympic Committee Sports Psychology Registry. Along the way, I kept bumping into Andy Ross, who had read and rejected my proposal in 2011. (On a side note, notice how I say "proposal" and not "me." Remember, the publishing of books is a business, and rejection is not personal.) When I had written my final proposal, I sent it out on a Tuesday in March 2013 to ten agents, including Andy. Several e-mailed me back right away—yet no word from Andy. However, the next morning, as I was driving into my San Francisco office, I got a phone call from Andy saying he wanted to represent me. Wow! My excitement level shot through the roof.

Since the day I went back to interviewing athletes in 2011, I've reimmersed myself in sports psychology and this book. My experiences, interviews, and research have convinced me that female athletes have different strengths and needs from male athletes. We are just different in the psychological and biological realms. I look forward to explaining and illustrating the basic core strengths of athletic females that are beneficial from knowing and understanding. The numerous illustrative stories depict the growth and needs of female athletes throughout the years. I hope readers will benefit from the wisdom of the girl and women athletes shared in the book. Thank you to all those who've helped me along the journey, which still continues.

ACKNOWLEDGMENTS

The saying "It takes a village" best describes the journey of this book. Without all the help from my relationships, including collaborating, bonding, intuitiveness, empathy, guidance, wisdom, and a "little bit of worry," this book would never have come to fruition. Each person provided me direction on the journey.

My heartfelt thanks go to the following individuals:

John Eric (JP) Poulson, my loving husband, has supported me through the process, beginning with the first written proposal in 1997.

Dr. Janice DeCovnick, my friend for thirty-two fruitful years, encouraged me from the germ of an idea in 1994 and went beyond the call of duty the night before I sent the manuscript to my publisher.

Ken Grace, my favorite coach, always shows a positive attitude, has inspired me as a sports psychologist and ultrarunner, and ultimately spreads sunshine to all those around him.

Linda Watanabee, a wonderful professional writer, showed her faith in my ability to write by inviting me to one of her advanced writing groups, and she knows how to have fun.

Cheryl Krauter and Terry Bowman, two fellow members of Linda's group, have continued as writing Facebook friends, sharing stories and optimism.

Brooke Warner, my book coach extraordinaire, guided me back to organization, outlining, and eventually writing a solid book proposal that led to my getting an agent and realizing a dream.

Andy Ross, despite rejecting my first proposal, had confidence and faith in my writing to give it another look and take me on as a client.

Krissa Lagos, my diligent editor, pushed swiftly through edits, especially at the end.

Pat Bracewell and Mary Jo McConahay have inspired and cheered me every moment of this past five years.

Dr. Susan Haradon has known and watched over me since I was a master's-level intern, as I grew into a full professional, and she recently conveyed to me how proud she is of me.

Jordan Rosenfeld helped get me back on track with my book idea and proposal.

Dr. Haleh Kashani lent me her expertise on eating disorders.

Dr. Mary Lamia frequently pushed me to get the book finished, which was always appreciated.

Dr. Patti (Katz) Chang, an old bike-riding friend, first suggested that I begin interviewing again and introduced me to Olympian Dr. Christine Thorburn.

Dr. Sharon Colgan, a fellow sports psychologist, pushed me to become a certified consultant through the Association of Applied Sports Psychology, which continues to open professional doors to this day.

Diana Illes Parker was responsible for introducing me to Sam Gash and Lisa Tamati, two extraordinary and pioneering women in finishing strong in multiday stage races.

Samantha Gash and Lisa Tamati have provided a continual source of inspiration.

Constance Hale taught me to omit using the verb "be" as much as possible.

Barbara Truax is my cheerleader extraordinaire, sharing friendship, writing wisdom, and her heart.

Steven Taylor Goldsberry shared his wisdom about finding a lively yet solid title.

David Meggyesy contributed generously in helping me connect with and interview extraordinary women.

Mike Spino—our mutual love of running bonded us immediately—provided me the opportunity to teach his sports-management class at Georgia State and to discuss men versus women in sports.

Juliette Goodrich and her mother, Paulette, assisted me in discovering the perfect title.

Robert Eichstaedt has helped me with computer issues and provided friendship throughout the multiple-year process of writing this book.

Dr. Catherine Main listened and encouraged when I hit rough spots. Although not an athlete herself, she has provided me with constant emotional support for all my athletic endeavors over the years.

Carmela Poulson provided faith, confidence, and support while I wrote the book.

Dean Steidinger taught me persistence, tenacity, and to have the toughest mind possible.

Frances Steidinger taught me the art of kindness and gave unconditional support through my entire master's and part of my PhD studies until she succumbed to breast cancer when I was only twenty-nine years old.

I also want to thank all of my book readers: Linda Aguilar, Dr. Janice DeCovnick, Maili Costa, Martha Cederstrom, Janice O'Grady, Danielle Schubert, and Stephanie Witt.

Most importantly, thanks to all girl and women athletes who inspire and teach us new lessons each and every day!

INTRODUCTION

Frequently moving around the country as an only (female) child taught me to get to know peoples' names, faces, and basic information quickly through my involvement in a wide variety of sports. What lacked was the opportunity to feel a sense of community or maintain best friends for very long. Certainly, swimming at age three, golfing at age five, and living on a real eastern Oregon working ranch and going on cattle drives at age ten built my self-confidence around knowing the mechanics of sports. It was exciting and fun and helped me become independent; yet interacting with other kids was sometimes difficult. My longing for a sense of community was ever present. As a teen (pre–Title IX), I found the meanness of other girls toward their "best friends" baffling and confusing. My southern mom's voice echoed, "Kill them with kindness," in my head, which didn't seem to work well. The worst coach of my life was my female high school tennis coach, who yelled criticism constantly and never said a nice word to me, only causing my game to get worse. I was thankful for badminton, which pushed me to play hard, and a number two ranking helped me feel confident, strong, and motivated, as did skiing the cornices and black diamonds with the boys. Qualifying to run in my high school's first girls' cross-country team was a dream, but mom soon cancelled that plan, as "it wasn't ladylike enough." My true desire rested in having athletic girlfriends who talked about relationships, shopping, and girly subjects. These were few and far between. Sports were a mainstay of validation as a person for me. Eventually, I took up running for exercising my first golden retriever and me.

In 1987, two years after finishing my PhD, something exciting happened as I prepared to run my first marathon in San Francisco. A friend, Peter Buttita, asked me if I wanted to be highlighted on the San Francisco Marathon show on NBC as a first-time marathoner. I jumped at the chance, and the experience felt fun and exhilarating. NBC filmed and interviewed me before, during, and after the race at the post-race party. The iconic Bob Costas, left with extra time to fill at the post-race gala, tried to interview me—young, blonde, pretty, and skinny as a rail—as if I were an elite runner. Most of my comments were, "Yes, I felt great!" at every mile he asked me about. As I was a first-timer, my enthusiasm got more pronounced with each question asked. The thrill of finishing your first marathon generally doesn't give rise to deep thought. A female psychologist friend of mine commented, "My only problem with you on television was you looked too good and made running a marathon sound too easy." The collaboration with the Fleet Feet Marina store "Marathon Training Program" had brought me camaraderie like I'd never felt before. Consequently, running evolved into my passion and meditation practice.

Upon moving to Marin County, California, in 1989 and immersing myself in running the trails on Mount Tam, I accidentally ran my first ultra. Getting permission from race director John Medinger (Tropical John), another running girlfriend, Donna, and I set out to run a double Dipsea while the Quad Dipsea was going on. When we finished the double on a crisp sunny November day, I asked John if we could keep going and register at the end. He said sure. The Quad was a low-key race back then on November 24, 1990, and we kept running through the clear, sunny day on the all up-or-down course and finished—but limped around the next week. Donna and I shared heartwarming bonding and fun. My "sisterhood in sports" was growing. Within the world of running/ultrarunning, I developed a whole repertoire of wonderful girlfriends whom I trained and raced with, including Lois, Barbara, Donna, Martha, Kathy, Janice, Kellie, Susanna, Debbie, Hazel, TJ, and Mary, and, boy, did we talk about relationships!

A few years prior to my entry into ultrarunning, a book came out titled *Women Who Love Too Much*, which immediately became a bestseller. Millions and millions of women were ecstatic about the book's message: women spend too much emotional time worrying and fretting about their relationships. As a young woman who had come to value her girlfriends, I was surprised by the sole focus on romantic relationships when we talked about most close relationships (romantic and otherwise), with some emotion attached, and certainly had fun engaging this way. As a few years passed in my private psychologist practice and noticing women in the worlds of ultrarunning and ride and tie (two people taking turns running and riding one horse), this focus on relationships seemed so commonplace that all these women and girls could not be sick or pathological. During that period, I further noticed how women, to a greater or lesser degree, consistently regarded their relationships more from an emotional perspective than men.

Given these three experiences, in my sports, professional (as a psychologist), and personal lives, my interest peaked about the role and effects of relationships in girls' and women's athletic lives. At this point, I began a new relationship with a man I met cycling; as I was developing the ability to compete in ultras, little did I know the relationship would erode my self-confidence and focus and cause me to feel alone again in my sporting abilities, eventually grinding down my training, racing time, and self-confidence. Winding my way out of this relationship, I decided to pursue the idea of writing a book and wrote my first serious proposal. That proposal was too subjective and so was promptly rejected by everyone who read it at the American Psychological Association Convention.

Shortly thereafter, in 1997, I began researching the role of relationships in women's athletics lives by interviewing forty brave ultrarunning women. My focus turned to a new love relationship. That man, JP, turned out to be my true love, and we married. He loves, admires, and respects strong female athletes and has encouraged me in sports and to bring these ideas over the years to pen and paper.

Sisterhood in Sports tells the stories of all kinds of female athletes in a variety of sports. Our natural tendencies to use talking as a primary form of communication, to make "best friends forever," to collaborate, to "tend and befriend" during stress, to intuit, to express empathy, to worry, and to seek fun in sports are all part and parcel of who we are as girl and woman athletes. These are our strengths grounded in both our minds and bodies. There are now dozens and dozens of studies showing how our brains and hormones operate quite differently from men's. In this book female athletes confirm that our intense emotions about relationships are part and parcel of who we are and describe how all of our relationships impact us. We enjoy and revel in our sisterhood. This emotional relationship focus is simply who we are, and we must embrace it in our sporting and personal lives and even in our work lives.

My parents used the motto "Kids should be seen and not heard." Until now, I was unaware that a good part of my motivation was to speak out and support female athletes. Seeing, hearing, and speaking are three imperatives for female athletes. As a female athlete, play your hardest, have fun in your sport, and don't be afraid to speak your mind about real and significant successes and injustices. After all, our primary strength comes from talking. As a remarkable and wise woman who's acted as a role model for many female athletes over the years and served as the grandmother of sports psychology, Dr. Carole Oglesby, strongly suggests, "Speak out. Even the biggest room needs a woman's voice."

I

SISTERHOOD IN SPORTS

Talking, Relationships, and the Unique Qualities of Female Athletes

Talking, talking, and more talking is what most girls, young and old, tend to enjoy—which is what makes talking and communicating so important when one is working with a female athlete. According to Dr. Louann Brizendine, the workings of the female brain influence how we communicate with one another in a significant way: we are hardwired to be more social and verbal than our male counterparts. Although there's been some dispute about the extent of this difference, there's no doubt about the fact that females tend to talk about relationships much more than males do—and this tendency extends to the athletic realm as well.[1]

Relationships are so vital to females that we handle stressful situations differently than do males. University of California, Los Angeles, professor Shelley E. Taylor conducted a groundbreaking study in 2000, revealing that women largely choose to protect their children or go to their friends for help in stressful situations. We do not just fight or take flight; we often choose to "tend and befriend" under stress. This instinct is clear in the sports world, where women on sports teams say that collaboration and camaraderie arise from talking and togetherness.

Studies of the female brain have revealed that "language is the glue that connects one female to another."[2] In focusing on female athletes' unique psychological and neurological functioning and better understanding how social connections are critical to their success, we can help these

athletes thrive. In this book, I offer an overview of how female athletes'
brains and minds impact their needs and strengths as individuals and in
relationships.

Some the unique qualities of the female brain include the significance
it places on emotional (intimate) connection, one-on-one friendships, empathy and intuition, positive peer-group collaboration and camaraderie,
and the desire for fun. Looking closely at neurological research findings,
we see substantial evidence supporting the idea that female athletes have
different needs from male athletes, and we will see that the female brain's
functioning plays a considerable role in these differences. Neurotransmitters from the brain, for example—such as oxytocin, which affects the
desire to bond and is found in much higher levels in the female than the
male brain—directly influence the behaviors female athletes display.

THE IMPORTANCE OF TALKING AND INTERPERSONAL COMMUNICATION

A primary concern in female athletes' lives is connection through intimate (emotional) relationships. These relationships consist of all types,
including (but not limited to) those with family members, friends, significant others, coaches, trainers, and teammates. Female athletes require
ongoing and regular spoken communication in their relationships in order
to feel connected. Psychological and physiological studies show that females are prone to be more social and verbal in their communication with
others than are males. Females and males may use the same number of
words in their interactions with others, but female dialogue generally
exhibits a greater focus on relationships and interpersonal communication. Relationship discussions, then, are of central importance to females,
be they athletic or nonathletic.

Time and time again in these chapters, you will see illustrations of the
role that talking plays in working with female athletes. This relationship
dialogue is one of the linchpins of effective communication with female
athletes. They are hardwired to engage in their relationships through language, and meeting that need is critical to their success.

In October 2012, I raised this debate about female versus male styles
of communication in a master's-level sports-management class at Georgia State where I was a guest speaker. That day, I spoke about the differ-

ing communication styles of male and female athletes. When I gave the class the opportunity to comment, a young man, Will, raised his hand immediately and described a recent exchange he'd had with his mother in which she asked him why he didn't talk about his feelings with his guy friends like she did with her girlfriends. He tried repeatedly to explain the differences between guy friends and girlfriends, he said, and she would have none of it. I told Will to tell his mother that I said he was right: there are social, cultural, psychological, and physiological factors that contribute to the different communication styles between males and females. These are not imagined differences.

Will wasn't the only member of the class who became engaged in the discussion. One young African American man, Ray, who was interning with a local pro sports team, spoke about his observations of the professional male athletes with whom he'd been spending intense periods, describing how the guys on the team were primarily focused on the mechanics of the game and how to get the best results and how they rarely, if ever, talked about their personal lives. Everything communicated was about game and strategy, he said, not feelings or personal relationships. He and other young men in the class even laughed about the idea of male athletes communicating their feelings to one another.

After Ray spoke, Tracy, one of the older and more mature women in the class, chimed in with her own perspective on females. Tracy thought that it was obvious that women are more likely than men to share personal stuff with their friends. "Women and men are totally different in their communication styles!" she said. She didn't need a scientific study to convince her of that fact.

Female athletes thrive when they receive thorough explanations and directions about how to execute new skills and why certain mental strategies are necessary. Daniella, a teenage softball pitcher I recently worked with on focus, concentration, and self-confidence, often came into my office for her sessions complaining that her coach didn't give her enough verbal explanations about how to improve. The coach—a burly, 6'3" man—would yell at her when she was pitching poorly at practice; he told her she was throwing too many balls and not enough strikes but never offered specific instructions about what she might do differently. Her shoulders would tighten, she would succumb to frustration, and her pitching would, if anything, get worse, not better.

Traditional coaching pushes athletes in impersonal and exceedingly aggressive ways, and it tends to be less effective with females than with males. Most women athletes respond better to collaboration than to opposition, and they are more likely to avoid conflict.[3]

I learned this lesson the hard way. A few years ago, I was negotiating a presentation to a group of Luna Chix (female athletes who raise money for breast cancer research) volunteer leaders at a nationwide Luna Chix summit held in Marin County, California. LaVonne, the coordinator at the time, and I agreed that I would focus on conflict resolution, so I worked numerous hours on a PowerPoint presentation in preparation for the event. When the day of the three-hour training arrived and I began to speak, however, none of the more than sixty-five women in the audience wanted anything to do with the subject. They only wanted to talk about motivation. I had to wing the entire training.

In 2012, I ran a three-day stage Nepalese Himalayan trail race (60K and 100K), and 2009 and 2010 USA Track & Field Ultrarunner of the Year Kami Semick happened to be there. She and I were discussing our mutual belief that women prioritize relationships over all else in their lives, and she said something that surprised me from a competitor of her level—that even though she enjoys being a front-runner, she sometimes misses the companionship of running with another runner and talking during races.

This comment took me by surprise because in thirty years of working with and being exposed to female athletes of all levels, I had never heard an elite woman runner express this sentiment. But Kami places a lot of value on her relationships—she is close to her family, and she often includes both her ten-year-old daughter and her husband in her exploits. Personal connections and deep discussions help her thrive. Watching her at the race, she spent a lot of time in intense one-on-one conversations with others. It makes sense, then, that she would miss such interactions when she's alone at the front of the pack.

Another family-oriented athlete, professional alpine skier Julia Mancuso, a gold (2006), double silver (2010), and bronze (2014) Olympic medalist, grew up in a large, extended Italian family full of talented female athletes who all supported and talked frequently to each other. She echoes this sentiment: "Just growing up with such strong females surrounding me, I always had a good self-image and outgoing personality. . . . As a younger athlete, I found it very important to have someone that believed in me. It helped me realize that I had something special and something worth fighting for." She credits her sister and father as her main inspirations.

Mancuso exemplifies the vital role of the relationship connection for female athletes. Her story illuminates how important having a strong and encouraging family group and close individual relationships is for women in sports. Female athletes put a strong value on having caring, supportive, and ongoing verbal interactions with friends, family, and the athletic personnel they work with. They need peer camaraderie—to talk with each other positively and regularly—in order to reach maximum team effort and results. Having a verbally and emotionally supportive crew, as Julia Mancuso does, makes all the difference for females competing and participating in sports.

THE IMPORTANCE OF RELATIONSHIPS

The story of Nike's former motto, "Just Do It," is an excellent example of the difference between female and male athletes. This motto may have worked for male athletes, but it was less effective for female athletes. Nike finally changed its motto in 2012; now it's "Find Your Greatness," which offers the positive element that women were missing in "Just Do It." The true motto for girls and women, however, the one that best exemplifies the female mentality, is "Relationships do it!"

Besides their sport itself, the subject most frequently discussed by female athletes is relationships. Both in and out of competition, female athletes like and rely on talking to communicate—and relationship information is a cornerstone of their conversations. In team sports, the development of peer-based collaboration and camaraderie is essential for the success of the team; relationships between teammates can directly affect an entire team's individual and overall athletic performance. For female athletes, relationship-focused discussions play an important role in the development of the camaraderie necessary to their success.

In the early 1990s, I competed with a local running club on the first women's ultrarunning team in Marin County. Certain team members were aware of and committed to being part of a team. At that time, the series only consisted of four races. Our team fully participated in all four. My desire to come through for my teammates was the motivator that helped me to hang in there throughout the series. There were five of us running, and three of us needed to finish for our team to place. In three of the four races, I was the first team member to finish, several times arriving half an hour to an hour ahead of the others.

When I left this team in 1994 and joined another, it was not because my previous team wasn't doing well—in fact, we won first place in the Pacific region's Ultrarunning Grand Prix Series, and I placed third in the Open Division in 1993—but because I felt underappreciated, even invisible, there. The club awards ceremony included one female member of the winning first-place ultrarunning team, and to my knowledge, she didn't even suggest that they invite the whole women's team or acknowledge that our success had been a group effort. I felt the interpersonal communication between certain team members was poor on that team, and for me it wasn't enough simply to win. I wanted the positive feedback and straightforward interactions that make it worth it to put forth that much effort. I felt the other club's team members, in contrast, were friendly and inclusive and that their interpersonal communications and reasonable appreciation for all the team's efforts were far better focused on the camaraderie that ultras encompass. As soon as I started running with them, I knew that making the switch to their club had been the right decision.

Even during a game or meet, women will talk about personal matters with their teammates if they are interested in connecting with them—and the feedback they get can affect their athletic performance. The way to get the best out of female athletes is to listen to and converse with them. Whether they are youth or adults, find out who they are and what they like. Do they have a significant other or spouse? How long have they been athletes? What other sports do they play? What are their passions? Does their family support their athletic endeavors? Female athletes appreciate it when others take an interest in all aspects of their lives, both personal and athletic. They want to know that people really care.

Makena, a seventeen-year-old volleyball player, had a strong relationship with her former coach, Liz. She said that Liz expressed care, concern, and commitment in their interactions, and she significantly helped Makena improve her game. Makena feels that her current coach, in contrast, "doesn't know how to coach." He's highly demanding and critical of the girls on the team. He rarely speaks with them on a personal level. Through Liz, Makena says, she learned to control her mental game and focus on having positive energy and thoughts, but this new coach has done nothing to help her advance further as an athlete. This is where her frustration remains.

I once watched a pro road cycling criterium—a race in which riders go around a circular course a designated number of times—and saw a perfect example of the ways in which female athletes may interact verbally with one another. At one point, three female racers were rounding a corner on their bikes, and one of them was aggressively working to cut in and cut off a couple of competitors. As they were rounding the corner, one woman yelled, "Stop cutting in!" The other firmly responded, "I'm not doing anything wrong!" The third woman rebuffed them both, saying, "Now, now, now, we'll have none of that!" I've never heard a male athlete make a remark like that during a race; in fact, in my experience most of the time they say nothing at all. Women are far more communicative, even in the heat of competition.

A second example of the active spoken communication that goes on between female athletes comes from my husband. He was in a road cycling race, and due to a series of mechanical issues, he had dropped back from his group and was riding just ahead of a women's paceline (cyclists riding along in a straight line, one behind the other). Technically, men are not supposed to ride in a paceline with the women, but the lead female rider rode up to him and remarked, "We've decided you can ride with us." He joined them, and for the rest of the race he listened, as they talked nonstop—mostly about relationship issues—until the race got serious. If it had been an all-male paceline, he said, they hardly would have spoken to one another at all—and certainly not about relationships.

Talking to others before, during, and after events doesn't always have a positive effect on female athletes, of course. For example, a young swimmer whom I worked with regarding her anxiety, Merrill, loved to talk with her girlfriends before meets, but when we took a closer look at this habit of hers, Merrill realized that too much talking with others just before her events made her anxious and affected her performance negatively. When she cut down on how much she interacted with others before her events and went to the blocks earlier, her performance improved.

Merrill also had an issue with a girl on her team, a rival who would make snotty remarks to her before competitions began. The comments often got under Merrill's skin—so much so that they interfered with her swimming outcomes. I had Merrill silently remind herself that she was a leader and a strong person when this happened so that she could ignore the girl's comments and focus on something positive instead; by mid-season, the other girl's words were no longer affecting Merrill. I also encouraged her to spend more time talking to her two good friends who were on her team when she did talk to other people during competitions. Stepping away from the negative and concentrating on positive thoughts helped Merrill to focus and compete better, and she also said that it made her feel confident that she could handle any interpersonal issues that she might come up against when she participated in swimming the following year at the collegiate level.

FEMALES VERSUS MALES: PRIMARY COMMUNICATION STYLES

In *The Female Brain*, Dr. Louann Brizendine establishes the significance of words to women, hypothesizing (based on her research) that women use about twenty thousand words per day, while men use only about seven thousand. Other studies dispute the number of words Dr. Brizendine suggests, but not the fact that women talk more about other people and relationships than men. Specifically Dr. Brizendine insists that "the circuits for social and verbal connection are more hardwired in the typical female brain." She goes on to assert that "some verbal areas of the brain are larger in women" than in men. Language and social connections, then, are critical to women's satisfaction and success in life; they are hardwired this way. Their brains absorb information more readily when they are spoken to, and their minds are therefore primed to communicate through the spoken word.[4]

Although there is some controversy over the exact number of words used by women versus men, experts seem to agree on one thing: women talk more about relationships than men do. Women's extra focus on relationships is part of who they are—part of their psychological and biological makeup—and it's something that comes into play powerfully with female athletes. Females need more ongoing positive rather than negative feedback to perform at their best as athletes; they respond better to clear, reasonable, and constructive communication than they do to harsh or supercritical comments.

Girls, especially when in their teens, will sit and talk for hours about relationships and how they feel about them. They need connections, spoken communication, one-on-one interactions with adult authority figures, and the support of those around them. They place value on learning personal things about the people they compete with. As a sports psychologist, I've watched girls and women compete for years, and I've seen firsthand how important relationships are to female athletes—how the attitudes of mothers, fathers, friends, siblings, teammates, and significant others can directly affect the performance outcomes of female athletes.

Women's acceptance and incorporation of their natural relational focus into their athletic lives is key to their building better self-confidence. As Judith V. Jordan and her coauthors write in *Women's Growth in Connection*, "For women especially, connections with others is central to psychological well-being. . . . Growth occurs in becoming a part of relationship rather than apart from relationship. Women's and girls' emotional, intellectual, physical, and spiritual growth can be enhanced or restrained by their relationships."[5]

Males, in contrast, generally communicate in more nonverbal and more cognitive ways, and they tend not to share personal details when in a group. Take, for example, a poker group profiled in the *New York Times* in August 2009. The nine men in the group had been playing together for years; yet they knew very little about each other. One or two had even gone through a divorce during the time that they'd been in the group, and none of the others knew about it. The article highlighted how differently men communicate from women, making the point that relationship and emotional discussions are simply not part of men's modus operandi.[6]

Another difference between male and female athletes is the fact that competition is a matter of course for males, but for women, it can pose a dilemma. A 2010 *Time* magazine article, "Girls versus Boys: The Perils of Competition," for example, made the argument—using studies conducted at California State University, Chico, and the University of Texas examining girls' and boys' view of competition—that boys find it easy to compete to win, but girls don't. Even after winning, in fact, girls express greater degrees of depression and loneliness following competition. This is because the need to focus on oneself for successful competition contradicts a woman's need to bond with others. World-class XTERRA triathlete Danelle Kabush says that focusing on the competitive part of sports was always less attractive to her as a young athlete than focusing on social interaction, and she has to work at maintaining a balance between the two. This is not uncommon for female athletes of all levels.[7]

This conflict between competing and collaborating is a source of struggle for many female athletes. Karen Brems, an Olympian and former directeur sportif for Webcor Women's Professional Cycling Team, describes a scene familiar to many female athletes: they lose a competition and then carry their disappointment around with them over time, talking and thinking about it frequently. Male athletes, in contrast, tend to leave their emotions behind; when an event is over, it's over. This difference isn't surprising when you consider that men have had centuries of learning how to be comfortable with sports-related competition and are more biologically programmed toward aggression (having ten times the testosterone level of women), whereas women, whose brains naturally struggle with conflict, have had only fifty or so years to adapt to athletic competition.

Female athletes still struggle with how to be competitive without sacrificing their relationships, though some have done so quite successfully. Serena and Venus Williams, for example, are positive role models for this: they have been fierce competitors over the years—both have been ranked number one in the world—yet have remained close friends throughout their illustrious careers. The duo of Kerri Walsh Jennings and Misty May-Treanor, Olympic multiple gold medalists and pro beach volleyball players, is another. They have certainly had their ups and downs in their partnership over the years. These girls even went jointly to a sports psychologist to work on their playing relationship before the last Olympic Games. Kerri described it like marriage counseling, commenting, "Absolutely. We're married. I have two amazing partners: My husband Casey and Misty. You gotta work through it. Sometimes you take things for granted. I've known her [Misty] for so long, but I don't know everything she's thinking. It's important to get on the same page." Both Kerri and Misty acknowledged that they benefited from the sessions. In 2012, they ended on a high note at the London Olympic Games, with their third gold medal and Misty exclaiming that they would be friends forever.[8]

FEMALES "TEND AND BEFRIEND"

In youth and adulthood, females thrive on verbal, supportive, and intimate relationships, both in their personal and athletic lives. The results of "Tend and Befriend," a 2000 study (mentioned earlier) led by Dr. Shelley E. Taylor that looked at women and stress, exemplify this fact. "Tend and Befriend" was the first study of its kind and magnitude to look at only women under stress. When they reviewed two hundred previous studies, Taylor and her colleagues found that women tend to speak to and join with others (especially children and girlfriends) when they are experiencing stress far more often than they engage in the fight-or-flight response. For the study's purposes, "tending" meant participating in nurturing activities designed to protect the self and offspring and to promote safety and reduce stress; "befriending," meanwhile, referred to the creation and maintenance of social networks that might aid in the tending process. [9]

Taylor's study further shows how pivotal a role emotional intimacy plays in women's lives and illuminates why verbal communication is so important for women in sports. When they experience "competitive stress," female athletes are best served by talking directly to others (except when they find that talking increases their stress and anxiety, in which case they need to engage in what I call "less stressful talking"— having a conversation with one or two calm friends or teammates about non-competition-related topics). Ongoing verbal communication and strong interpersonal relationships, therefore, are integral to the success of females in training and competition.

Tending and befriending plays out in an important way for women in sports. Many women who competed in the 2012 Olympic Games and Olympic trials described the importance of training partners in interviews, for example—and you can bet that their interactions with those partners included conversations about relationships. In striving to represent the United States in the 2008 Summer Olympics, Erin Maxwell and Isabelle Kinsolving put on a gallant campaign to meet this goal. These two female sailors worked in perfect harmony on a 4.7-meter boat in order to cross the finish line first at the 2008 World Championships in Australia. Maxwell and Kinsolving worked intensely and pushed themselves to their absolute maximum in order to win—but their hard work only came to fruition because of their strong spoken communication and willingness to work together.

Racing the Planet's annual 4 Deserts Race Series consists of the Atacama Crossing in Chile, the Gobi March in China, the Sahara Race in Egypt, and the Last Desert in Antarctica. Samantha Gash was not a professional runner; she was a law student and law clerk and an absolute newcomer to ultrarunning. She had just completed her first marathon prior to running her first six-day race. Still, she decided to participate in the Atacama run—partnering with a new friend, Andrea Bassman (a woman from Tahoe and the Bay Area), for the race—and they had a good experience doing it. Following the race, Samantha kept in touch with Jen Steinman, who was filming a documentary movie on the 4 Deserts races, and at some point Samantha decided to become the first woman to complete the 4 Deserts series.

Samantha arrived at the Gobi March only to discover that her ultrarunning idol, Lisa Tamati—a well-known ultrarunner in Australia and a nationally known athlete in New Zealand—was there. Lisa enjoys celebrity status in New Zealand. Samantha and Lisa struck up a conversation about Lisa's autobiography, *Running Hot*, and the 2,200K run across New Zealand Lisa had recently done to raise money for two children's charities. On the first day of the race, Lisa and Samantha discovered that they had similar pacing—they kept crossing paths throughout the day—and on the fifth day of the race (which was a 100K stage), Lisa asked Samantha to run with her. According to Jen Steinman (director of *Desert Runners*), "Samantha was flattered to have Lisa ask her." In these multi-day stage races it's a common occurrence for the racers to plan to run together, especially on the longer 100K day at the end, but there are not many female front-runners to run with. This running together is done for safety, security, and mental support. During the Gobi March, they ran in a region of conflict between the Wen and Han Chinese. The police presence was ever felt.

Sam and Lisa helped each other through emotional highs and lows. They ran along chatting, although they were racing, and got to know each other well. Collaboration and camaraderie were essential to the process. They took turns crying and building each other up. They were seen leaving a checkpoint holding hands and constantly passed other racers all day and night in the steady ultrarunners shuffle. Jen observed, "Lisa was racing but Samantha was in it to run. Lisa taught Samantha how to race. Both accomplished so much more together than they would have individually." They ran as BFFs.

Samantha and Lisa talked about one particularly funny incident. They were lost in the desert at night, desperately looking for disappearing glow sticks with only headlamps to guide them, and the girls' water supply was running low. They were thirsty and worried. Finally, they came across a spring with a big wooden trough full of water. Both girls started crying, threw their packs down, and dove in head first with their headlights still on and only their bums sticking out. What a sight! Next thing Lisa knew, she turned around to see Samantha's bum sticking straight in her face. Samantha was taking a pee. According to Lisa, the whole bloody mess seemed so hilarious, they started cracking up and laughing hysterically. They could barely stop laughing. Eventually, they gathered their composure and began running again. At the end of the race were huge sand dunes. Here, they crawled and, using their headlamps, hoped to stay on the course lit only by glow sticks. Eventually, they ran separately to the finish. Lisa landed second-place female and twentieth place overall in the Gobi March. Samantha came in first in her age group and twenty-eighth overall in only her second six-day stage race.

Samantha also went on to become the youngest and first woman to complete the 4 Deserts Race Series. What these two women achieved running these ultras shows us what females need to form close bonds in sports. They chatted, formed a solid one-on-one relationship, shared all types of emotions (from laughter to tears), collaborated, and had a whole pile of fun. Plus, their hard work, both physical and mental, helped bring them success in their athletic endeavors. They remain close running friends today.

Bonding between young female athletes is equally important as it is for adult women. With teenage girls, tending and befriending is everything. They gather, gossip, and giggle with their friends—endlessly at times—and they often have a hard time putting their focus on sports above their focus on friends and dating. Young female athletes who start sports early and maintain participation as part of their lifestyle, however, are more likely to overcome the potential distractions and stick with their athletic pursuits.

According to the Wilson Report (1988), "Parents' own behavior influences their daughters, since parents who play tend to have daughters who play—70 percent of daughters who currently participate have parents who also engage in sports or fitness activities."[10]

One of these young women whose parent and brothers shared sports with her is Terry, a tall, lanky blonde with a casual manner who is a member of a local powerhouse mountain bike team. Terry names her number one influence as her mother. "Mom is my cheerleader. My mom and I mountain bike for fun," she explains. In fact, her whole family (her mother and her two brothers) is outdoorsy: they all camp, hike, and ride mountain bikes together.

Whereas Terry's family has always been very supportive, however, her friends have not. Her involvement in athletics has hindered her relationships at times. This is not uncommon; peers and significant others often pressure teenage female athletes to drop out of sports in order to hang out with them more, a phenomenon the Wilson Report refers to as the "puberty barrier."[11] Terry's family was there for her, but she struggled with maintaining her relationships with her nonathletic female friends during high school because they just didn't understand the amount of time her team and training took. Her solution was to develop a group of friends who were all involved in competitive sports—a decision made by many girls who start playing sports at young ages.

ATHLETICS AND THE UNIQUE BRAINS OF FEMALES

Hormones in our brains directly influence our behavior. For females, this has a profound impact on our athletic lives. In the 1990s, the government (through the National Institutes of Health [NIH] Revitalization Act of 1993) started requiring that all NIH-funded research studies include females. Since then, there has been extensive research into the workings of the female and male brains, especially through the use of brain scans. A number of our behaviors can be explained by the function of the brain. Hormones like oxytocin, estrogen, and dopamine, for example, are all found in higher levels in the female than the male brain. They have been shown to contribute to women's desire for bonding and tendency to make relationships all-important in their lives. Dopamine directly relates to pleasure and motivation, high oxytocin levels push females toward a wish for intimacy, and estrogen guides us on a daily basis toward deeper emotional intimacy.[12]

Since the publication of Dr. Louann Brizendine's *The Female Brain* in 2006, we have seen amazing advances in our understanding of how the female brain works through dozens of studies that support the relevance of many of her assertions, including her claim that "maintaining the relationship at all costs is the female brain's goal."[13] The simple fact, which Brizendine so clearly expresses, is that there is no unisex brain. Female and male athletes do not think or act exactly alike. Our brains are physiologically different, and this difference directly affects our actions and our requirements for success. When under extreme stress and duress (as is often the case in training and competition), female athletes look to their relationships for assistance.

Female athletes are driven, first and foremost, to hang on to their relationships. They experience emotional connections. This biological and psychological compulsion to connect with others often creates a special dilemma for teen female athletes being pressured to drop out of sports by their peers. The conflict becomes friends and boyfriends versus sports, and it's difficult for females to make that choice. Enough pressure from nonathletic friends can create what I term "the relationship versus sport dilemma."

One of my former clients, a young female swimmer named Sarah, had a mother who did not encourage her to have other teammates as friends. In fact, she taught Sarah to think that she was better than all her teammates—to look at other swimmers in her event only as competitors, never as friends. Because of this, Sarah's only friends were not athletes, and they constantly pressured her to spend less time swimming and more time with them. When I realized the true dynamics of the situation and suggested working with Sarah and her mother together, Sarah's mother pulled Sarah out of our sessions altogether. If she had allowed us to continue to work together, I would have encouraged Sarah to befriend some of her teammates. I often suggest to both my teenage and adult female athlete clients who are looking for new friendships or a romantic relationship to focus on other athletes.

Dr. Brizendine and other researchers often talk about the ways in which the specific workings of the female brain directly impact female athletes. The most predominant features of the female brain are language, intimacy through emotion (relationships), intuition, empathy, collaboration, self-control, a bit of worry, discomfort with conflict, and a different way of expressing aggression.[14] As Dr. David Geary of the University of Missouri puts it, "Females use language more when they compete."[15]

The language function in women actually crosses over onto both sides of the brain, which helps to explain why female athletes have such a need for strong verbal communication. Language helps female athletes understand their sport better. In my office, I frequently hear complaints from female athletes about the lack of thorough explanations from coaches and others when they are struggling with an aspect of their sport. Daniella, the teenage softball player I talked about earlier in this chapter, is not the only female client I've had who has told me that her coach's yelling and nonspecific criticism not only don't help her but confused her further.

Susie, a teenage basketball player I worked with, had a problem similar to Daniella's—except her trouble was with her dad. He attended most of her games, but his yelling and criticism were hurting her morale and performance. Once she got comfortable enough to speak with him about the issue, they were able to discuss her needs at games in a constructive way and improve their relationship. Unfortunately, Daniella, even with assistance from her mom, was unable to get her needs met with her high school coach, even after she communicated them to him. Ultimately, Daniella's mom hired private coaches who were particularly helpful and understood how to communicate with Daniella and address her needs.

Strikingly, this issue of intimacy with females creates the emotional foundation for their relationships. Their investment at a deeper emotional level contributes to their connections and success—which is perfectly exemplified by the relationship between Kerri Walsh Jennings and Misty May-Treanor. Male athletes' conversations and connections tend to be primarily cognitive and activity based, but female athletes focus their attention and discussions on their relationships. This type of bonding is strongly affected by the neurotransmitters oxytocin, estrogen, and dopamine. These differences in the brain makeup of women and men make women generally more skilled at recognizing and empathizing with the emotions of other people. As Dr. Ruben Gur, a neurologist at the University of Pennsylvania, asserts, "Women are faster and more accurate with identifying their emotions."[16]

In an extensive study of twenty-six thousand women and men, well-known (albeit controversial) neuropsychiatrist Dr. Daniel Amen compared women's and men's brain activity through the use of MRIs (brain scans) and SPECT scans (which monitor blood flow and activity levels), and he discovered that females showed more activity in seventy of the eighty areas measured. In his book *Unleash the Power of the Female*

Brain, Dr. Amen talks about its strengths. In particular, he focuses on the five main strengths of the female brain that stand out the most in his research: intuition, empathy, collaboration, self-control, and a little worry. Not all scientists agree with Dr. Amen, but they do agree that neuroimaging will be a critical part of future research—and it's clear that studies of the brain can offer us an even broader understanding of female athletes' brains in terms of needs and motivations.

ALL ABOUT FEMALE ATHLETES

Females of all ages love to talk. The content of their talking often includes a focus on relationships. These are two important facts to remember when dealing with female athletes of any age, whether they are at the youth, collegiate, pro, or Olympic level. You'll find no better example of this than the keynote speech that Tony DiCicco, head coach of the 1996 gold-medal-winning women's soccer team, gave at the 2012 Association of Applied Sports Psychology Conference. In the speech, DiCicco described an interaction that he had with Mia Hamm before the 1996 Olympics. At one point, DiCicco explained, Hamm asked to speak to him in private.

"Coach, are you mad at us?" Hamm asked. "Are we in danger of getting cut?"

"No," DiCicco replied surprised.

"Then quit yelling at us!" Hamm said.

DiCicco took heed, realizing that if he simply spoke to his athletes, they would listen to him. He still pushed them hard to perform well and achieve their Olympic dream, of course—but he recognized that his athletes needed to be encouraged and to feel free to speak with their coaches and with each other, if they were going to succeed. It's time that we all, like DiCicco, recognize that female athletes are hardwired to speak more, focus their attention on relationships in an emotional way, and socialize. This is a vital part of understanding how female athletes tick.

We know that talking, talking, and talking some more about relationships is what females do. As you might recall from earlier in this chapter, the language function is so predominant in the female brain that it operates on both the left and right side. We also know that this talking serves a need female athletes have to feel connected to others—and with positive spoken communication, female athletes are more likely to perform at their best. If we're not feeling good, we're more likely to tank.

Male athletes tend to approach their sport as a test of mastery over themselves and their competitors. They don't need the spoken affirmation that female athletes do. Young competitive female athletes are often more interested in the social aspects of their lives, however—which means that social interaction and spoken communication are of the highest priority for those working with them. But all female athletes, young and mature alike, look to their social networks for support in times of stress; when we are under pressure, we are more likely to try to find someone to speak with about it than male athletes are. Social networking for female athletes is essential. We find our value in talking and connecting with others, both in and out of sports. Our brains work for us through our relationships and bonding, emotions, empathy, intuition, collaboration, self-control, appropriate worry, and desire for fun.

TEN MENTAL STRATEGIES FOR FEMALE ATHLETES

1. Use your talking talents to your advantage.
2. Develop friendships with other female athletes you can confide in.
3. Remember that "relationship dialogue" is a cornerstone of your success.
4. When under stress, "tend and befriend."
5. Find friends who support and listen to you about your sport.
6. Look for men or women who are also athletic when seeking a romantic relationship.
7. Ask for detailed and specific verbal explanations about new sport techniques.
8. If you are a member of a team, work on being inclusive with all team members.
9. Remember your brain's strengths include talking, relationships and bonding, collaborating, intuiting, feeling for others, and the desire to have fun!
10. Remember the true female athlete's motto: Relationships do it!

2

BEST FRIENDS FOREVER

Teenage Trials and Building Long-Lasting Friendships

"**B**est friends forever" is the current phrase for depicting close female relationships, especially in the teenage years. Teenage girls thrive—especially as athletes—when they have best friends. Just the other day, I held a sports psychology workshop for female teen athletes. Three moms (one an athlete), a coach/athlete, and five teens showed up. I was impressed at the openness exhibited by everyone involved. Both the teens and the adults wanted to learn about and discuss sports psychology; yet they also wanted to understand each other on a more personal level. The group tried out suggestions, such as visualization in the outdoors, and discussed viewpoints about varying techniques in sports psychology, along with focusing on a positive attitude. We enjoyed a lot of laughter. The camaraderie and fun we experienced that night is illustrative of the kind of information, both personal and sports specific, shared when girls and women interested in athletics gather together in a group. Before the night was over, strong group camaraderie had been created: everyone there was working to support and talk to one another.

Girls' teenage friendships depend heavily on the relationships around them—and this is especially true for athletic girls. Best friends are important to females, especially during our teen years. With about one in three high school girls participating and competing in high school sports, as opposed to half of all high school boys, we need to pay attention to the differences and similarities between the two sexes. In 2009, *Time* magazine ran an article titled "Why Girls Have BFFs and Boys Hang Out in Packs" that looked at research by the National Institute of Mental Health on the brain differences between girls and boys that impact their social orientation. Brain scans taken during the study showed that, when they are given social choices, the social centers of young girls' brains showed greater activity than those of boys.

The thirty-four girls and boys participating in the study, who ranged in age from eight to seventeen, were shown photos of boys and girls and asked to rate those photos on a scale from "not interested" to "very interested." They told the kids that they would arrange for them to chat online with the kids they liked; when they brought them back together at a later date, they asked them to guess which of the kids in the photographs also wanted to chat with them and ran a functional magnetic resonance imaging (fMRI) scan on the kids while they did so. The scans showed that parts of the girls' brains became more active at the prospect of meeting someone new, whereas the boys' brains showed no such increase in activity. The girls were especially disappointed when they found out the photos only showed actors or actresses and they would not actually be chatting with them.[1]

BEST FRIENDS AND GIRLS: TEEN FRIENDSHIPS

In the teen years, there is a strong desire for cooperation and connection—and females primarily connect through talking and sharing the intimate details of their lives. Imagine, today over 3.2 million girls in the United States play high school sports. They relate and connect in an emotional way. This verbal bonding is essential to girls in sports and life. Words and the details they express solidify girls' connections with others. "Half of all girls who participate in some kind of sport experience higher than average levels of self-esteem and less depression."[2] Their talking may help them to be less inclined toward depression. Without it, they cannot thrive—which is why teenage female athletes need best friends who support their involvement in sports, whether their best friends are athletic or not.

According to the Women's Sports Foundation, fourteen-year-old girls drop out of sports at twice the rate of fourteen-year-old boys. Although this percentage has progressed from previous years, there is still improvement to make. Before their teenage years, girls look more to their parents and siblings for support; around age thirteen or fourteen, however, peers and boyfriends become even more important. Without like-minded male and female friends, teenage athletic girls can get pulled in a multitude of directions. Peers and boyfriends make up several of the major reasons for teenage girls dropping out of sports. Sports take a major time commitment, and teenage female athletes often have to miss out on social opportunities. This sacrifice can create ambivalence about their sport, especially if they don't have athletic friends. This happens less frequently in places where there is tremendous emphasis on youth sports, but even then it still occurs. [3]

With the increasing number of younger girls participating in competitive sports, it is crucial that we encourage our athletic girls to make friends who are also athletic and to maintain those friendships throughout junior high and high school. If we want our girls to participate in sports, we need to encourage them to have friends who will support that participation.

Years ago, working with a talented thirteen-year-old Marin County girl teen swimmer, I discovered she had mixed feelings when it came to her inability to do more social activities. She swam for both a high school and a club team. Her nonathletic friends questioned why she was so busy all the time with swimming. The conflict was between swimming, other sports, and nonathletic social activities. She worked with me and improved her performance skills but struggled with her dilemma. She lacked athletic girlfriends, which contributed to the problem. Her overly controlling mother did not help the situation. Eventually, her mother pulled her out of work with me when I suggested that she attend some sessions with her daughter. This is just one example of when a teenage girl got help for performance but was still at risk of dropping out of swimming.

A contrasting example is Kristy Wentzel, who rowed for the Marin Rowing Association during her teen years. Her German father, Jochen, played field hockey for Germany in the Pan American Games when he was younger, her mother is a runner and rower, and her three younger sisters, Megan, Carrie, and Amy, all play volleyball competitively. Amy also swims. The girls were all raised in Marin County, California, which is a haven for elite athletes. In Kristy's family, everyone is expected to show up when someone has a sporting competition. The girls in this family experienced support from both family and friends.

In 2009, Kristy was part of the Junior National USA Team that won the World Rowing Junior Championship against France on the 8+ boat. The night before the competition, she says, she was "flipping out," but her teammates helped her calm down by surrounding her and reminding her that she had worked hard and deserved to be on the boat and that they were all equally nervous about the race. In other words, she was not alone. This feedback and support, Kristy says, helped her to perform her best the next day in the race against France in which they were victorious.

The fact that Kristy is friendship oriented throughout her sports and academic career contributes greatly to her success as an athlete. In high school, she made woven friendship bracelets in her team colors for both her Marin Rowing teammates (red, black, and white) and her Junior National teammates (red, white, and blue), for example. This may seem like a small gesture, but it is emblematic of the support Kristy gave her teammates throughout training and competing—and judging by her achievements, that success came back to her in spades.

According to the Women's Sports Foundation, there is a positive and strong connection between participation in high school sports and academic achievement for all youth, but especially for girls. Kristy is a gleaming example of this: after high school, she went on to attend and row for Stanford.

According to a 2007 study by Kelly P. Troutman and Mikaela J. Dufur, females who participate in high school sports are also more likely to complete college than those who do not participate in sports.[4] This is partly because teenage girls who participate and compete in sports learn about setting goals and objectives and striving to accomplish them through structure. Teen female athletes also benefit from having girl-friends who are motivated to set their own goals and objectives, whether or not they are sports related. Nonathletic friends can be just as positive an influence as athletic friends for young female athletes, as long as they are understanding and supportive of the time and dedication competitive sports require. Sports are a common focus for teenage athletes to bond with friends over, but that doesn't mean they can't also bond with other friends on an emotional basis. According to a Women's Sports Foundation fact sheet about teen girls in sport, "Participation on an athletic team in high school can increase a girl's chance of graduating by 41% . . . as well as increase self-confidence, self-esteem and problem-solving skills."[5]

Mackinzie Stanley, a competitive runner and mountain biker in high school, valued and benefited from the support during high school she received when she had two hip replacements. She fought hard in rehab. It took day after day of consistent rehabilitation for her to return to competitive form. She emphasized, "My support system made all the difference, including family and teammates at Drake High School [in San Anselmo, California]." She is a young woman who views the world optimistically, even with her reserved manner. In 2011, she gave an inspirational keynote at an Annual NorCal (Northern California) Mountain Biking banquet in Mill Valley, California, describing her experience. She is just one of many women who prefer to bond by talking about positive topics and outcomes and supporting each other mentally and physically. Mackinzie, also a former Whole Athlete Mountain Bike Racing girls' team member, summed it up nicely: "Being with a whole bunch of friends and fellow athletes helped keep the atmosphere light and fun, even right before a race, and it helped keep down the nerves. Plus, we had each other to lean on for help and encouragement."

Nonathletic friends can be just as positive an influence as athletic friends for young female athletes, as long as they are understanding and supportive of the time and dedication competitive sports require. However, they can also be a negative influence if they discourage the intensity of commitment that competitive sports often demand. A frequent problem is for nonathletic girlfriends to pressure their friends to come out and party, even when they have athletics events the following morning.

When speaking to three groups of teenage female basketball players (varsity, junior varsity, and freshman teams), I observed the close relationships among them. I sat at a table with each group to discuss the basic principles of sports psychology; in each group, the girls sat near their best friends and were vocally supportive of one another. They even gave each other feedback about better ways to provide support when one player was being critical of some of the younger, more inexperienced, players. "You would help us more if you tried to take more shots at the rim when you are open," one freshman player said. "That would be better than just yelling about what we're doing wrong and criticizing us."

During my meeting with the group, I encouraged the three seniors who had been playing the longest to lead their teammates by using positive communication. Apparently, the previous team had worked together well, but this team was having trouble coming together. As I emphasized the need for a more positive approach and the importance of fun, the girls began to give me direct eye contact and nod in agreement. After our short time together, the coach told me that she had learned a lot during the session. The message even got through to the most critical girl, Melody; when the session ended, she asked, "When are we going to do this again?"

HOW BEST FRIENDS HELP IN SPORTS AND LIFE

Female athletes are talkers and listeners. They like nothing more than to sit down face-to-face and have a chat with someone. Often, they just want to be heard. Women bond much more through emotional expression. They want others to know about and be interested in them personally. Close girlfriends fulfill this desire—which is why the lives of female athletes, like those of all women, are enriched by having best girlfriends.

Teen girls are just learning to compete against each other in friendlier ways and still call each other best friends. This represents a new era when girls can play sports with each other and remain friends. Back in 2009, two teen track-and-field runners in Arizona often had times within fractions of each other, yet remained best friends off the track. Jessica Tonn and Sarah Penny often ran neck in neck, with Tonn pulling slightly ahead in their final season in high school. Sarah watched those tapes to pump her up. Their friendly rivalry helped each other strive for more. They both went off to college with track-and-field scholarships, Jessica at Stanford and Sarah at the University of Oregon.[6]

Jessica, in a recent video interview after hitting a 9.10 3K personal record (PR) in the 2013 University of Washington January meet, was thrilled with the outcome. She appeared just as optimistic as she had as a teen. She described running as fun and perfect. She commented, "Weird, running is fun. I've only been doing it for a decade." Hopefully, this is how more teen girls in sport can evolve more positive attitudes toward sport participation, since fun is so important to females in general.[7]

These high school friendships can carry on into adult life. My friend DeDe and I have enjoyed a friendship since high school. We were both devoted backpackers and snow skiers. In high school and in the years that followed, we skied many mountains together. We actually belonged to a Girl Scout troop in high school whose main activity was taking its members on numerous backpack trips, mainly in Southern California. So DeDe and I spent intense periods in the wilderness where we literally watched each other's back. We were both heavily involved in school activities as well. On different months, we were both named "Girl of the Month" and were honored by the La Habra Women's Club for our leadership and accomplishments in high school. As adults, we continued to go on skiing trips together. Eventually, I became extremely interested in running races, evolved into ultrarunning, and became competitive. DeDe didn't share my interest in this particular area of athletics, but our friendship has stretched on from then until today. We're both closing in on sixty now, but our friendship is strong and has endured the passage of time.

In 1993, DeDe helped me take on one of the harder sporting events I've ever competed in: the Western States 100-Mile Endurance Run. DeDe had never even been to an ultrarunning event (a race over 26.2 miles) before, but she enthusiastically jumped in with both feet to help. It was just like high school: she flew north from San Diego, drove me to Tahoe two days before the race started, put up with my self-doubt and pre-race jitters, and made ten peanut butter and jelly sandwiches on sourdough bread for me to eat at the aid stations placed along the race course—and when I was fully thrashed after the race, she drove me back to the Bay Area. And she did it all without sleeping for thirty-eight hours.

DeDe was my crew boss at the race, along with two other supportive and enduring crew members, Lisa and Mike Locati. I approached the race optimistic that I might achieve my goal of finishing in under twenty-four hours. Despite this, I got so nervous the day before the race, talking fast and pacing back and forth, that I accidentally put the shoes I'd inserted my orthotics into in the mile seventy-eight aid station drop bag, which we'd given to another crew member. I didn't discover that they were missing until the morning of the race, a little before the 4 a.m. start. While I panicked, DeDe kept a level head: she assigned a male crew member to track them down and bring them back ASAP. In the meantime, another friend of mine who was there, Cheryl, lent me her orthotics on the spur of the moment. It was a nice thought, but they were tight and rubbed against the bottom of my feet. By mile twenty, my feet were two-thirds blistered on the bottom. My goal for running the race in under twenty-four hours went straight out the door.

On top of that, the mass start of the race takes you over Immigrant Pass in Tahoe, which meant we spent the first twenty miles of the race running in snow. For me, it was a process of running and falling on my butt, running and falling on my butt—to the point that the other runners coined a term for it, calling it my "fall, butt, and run" method.

The Western States trail goes through a series of canyons at one point; that year, the temperatures got up to 112 degrees in some of the canyons. It was truly a survivalist event, and I was determined to be a survivor, no matter what lay ahead. At the Last Chance (mile 43.3) aid station, I finally sat down with the medical personnel on staff and allowed them to dress my feet with Second Skin (a thick, cushioned sheet of antiseptic) to make the miles ahead more bearable—but still, no orthotics appeared.

On Michigan Bluff, at mile fifty-six, I saw what I'd been looking for: DeDe standing there holding up my orthotics. It had taken her until then to find the male crew member sent out to retrieve my orthotics that morning. By then, it was late afternoon, and she had spotted my running shoes sitting on the dashboard of the crew guy's small Toyota truck, baking in the hot sun at Foresthill (mile sixty-two). She located him in the crowd, had him unlock the truck, grabbed the orthotics, and stepped on the gas to drive them to me. I'd never been so happy to see DeDe as I was in that moment, slowly running up the hill toward her. I put my orthotics in my shoes immediately, and even though my feet were massively blistered, they still felt like a relief.

After that I regrouped and ran on to Foresthill, where DeDe greeted me once again. In addition to DeDe, I had Lisa, my pacer, who expressed continual words of encouragement and support the whole length of the twenty miles that she was pacing. Her husband, Mike, was present as well and cheering me on. She said nothing when she saw the bottom of my raw and blistered feet after the river crossing at mile seventy-eight, but she later confessed to me that when she saw them, she knew I was running on sheer will.

When Lisa's twenty miles were up, a male friend of mine, David, took over, helped straighten my mind out when it became confused, and paced me into the finish. We ran/walked up to Robey Point (mile 98.5) together, and we soon landed back on the road with just one mile left to go. I'd had a rough day, but I knew I was going to cross the finish line. As we made our way to the end, one of my Tamalpa running club friends yelled, "We gave up on you hours ago!" My response: "Never give up on me—I'm a finisher!" And it's true—but I couldn't have done it without the help of my crew and friends, especially my old friend (DeDe) from high school.

THE IMPACT OF SPORTS AND SOCIALIZING

In the teen years, the desire for cooperation and connection reigns supreme. Without best friends who support their involvement in sports, teenage female athletes do not thrive, and they often stop playing sports altogether. These teen athletes, then, depend upon their best friends forever (BFFs) to help them stay on track with their athletic pursuits.

The teenage years are a time when the mean girls emerge. These are the girls who can't be trusted and disrupt a group readily. The mean girl teens are catty, incessantly talking behind each other's back in unkind ways. During this time, cliques form, and not everybody is allowed in. Even "best friends" may talk behind your back. Teens need to realize that girls who do this are not best friends, especially in sport. When cliques form within a sports team, which they inevitably will, disruptive girls may need to be taken aside and talked to. Even if great players on the team, they may need to be benched during games, pulled out of events, and so forth. Cliques may hurt or help a team. Ignoring the mean girls will not make them go away. Hopefully, if the positive girls are placed in the forefront, their upbeat energy will direct the team and best friends to rally their playing together. Empowering multiple team members by giving them tasks to lead (such as rallying teammates during different times in a game) helps the girls to bond. Sports provide a venue for girls to learn about helping one another and watching each other's back.

Sports participation helps teenage girls build the foundation for future success. The Women's Sports Foundation has discovered that in Fortune 500 companies, 80 percent of female CEOs say they participated in sports in their youth. But the teenage years tend to be a tumultuous time in a girl's life. Socializing is the all-important activity, and nonathletic friends and boyfriends often take girls away from sports. Add peer pressure into the mix, and we see how the teenage athlete can struggle to fit in socially. Even Danelle Kabush, a pro XTERRA triathlete, says that when she was a teen, her interest was primarily in the social aspects of sports, not the competition.

With the increasing participation of younger girls in competitive sports, we must encourage our athletic girls to make sports-playing friends and maintain those friendships through junior high and high school. Best friends come in a variety of forms—from sisters to coaches to fellow teammates—but whatever shape they take, they are key to helping teens discover the joy of sports and the fun of competition.

TEENAGE GIRLS IN GROUPS AND ON TEAMS

Girls often hang as a group, talking about relationships in life and sport. Female athletes on teams tend to relate to one another as peers, talking about their personal lives and confiding in one another. Male athletes, in contrast, tend to have a top-down approach, with one guy as the top dog and the other team members lining up behind him in a more hierarchical order. This difference is due in part to the more collaborative nature of females. And coaches often say they've noticed this difference in the female athletes they work with.

In team sports (such as basketball, volleyball, and soccer), bonding is essential for effective teamwork and camaraderie. On girls' teams, team members typically know more personal details about one another than members of a boys' team would, which may or may not help them bond. The attitudes and emotions that team members outwardly display and the cliques they form can have a huge impact on how the team performs. Teenage girls, for instance, band together in small groups and usually have best friends. If a team lacks this ingredient of team camaraderie, or if some members on the team are being excluded, team-building activities are necessary. Ultimately, many working parts—parents, siblings, friends, coaches, boyfriends, girlfriends, and the girls themselves—impact a team. Emotional closeness and team excitement bring about a sense of collaboration and allow the girls to have fun together.

I recently worked with San Rafael High's Varsity Girls' Basketball Team. They clearly needed a different and fresh perspective. Before I met with the girls, their head coach, C.J. Healy, shared with me that the girls had lost every game in the season but had a chance (a slim one) of winning a game that week. When I spoke with the girls the night before the game, I talked to them in a positive manner about persistence, hard work, and team camaraderie. Initially, they all seemed reticent, so I randomly selected girls from the group and asked them questions about themselves and their strengths as players. When asked how motivated they were on a scale of one to ten, one team member, Selena, yelled out, "Twenty-five!" This simple, enthusiastic comment spurred on the other girls to participate more in the discussion. Quickly, I asked the other team members what it would take for all of them to be motivated like Selena to win the next game. They immediately fired back factors that I had mentioned during my talk: focus, wanting to win, playing better, getting excited, and being persistent. By the end of our talk, the girls were all engaging more with one another. I encouraged them all to remember the thoughts we'd just discussed during their game the next day, and they appeared to leave the session with a more positive attitude than they had first started with.

The next day, I sent a brief e-mail to the girls' coach, C. J., asking her to let me know how they had done. Her response: "We won! We won by a lot! The girls were on fire!" She went on about the miraculous transformation and how they had won by thirty-five points. The girls had persisted, gained a different perspective, and used the power of being positive to work together with momentum and camaraderie. They not only won—they smoked the other team. In doing so, they displayed their strength as a team and ended their season on a high note, more connected and bonded than ever before.

The performance of these girls left little doubt in my mind about the importance of being positive and connected as players. When I first arrived to speak to the team, the male assistant coaches looked at me with apparent skepticism (though they did appear more open after I met with the girls). And the head coach, C.J., expressed almost disbelief, yet elation, when the girls played like a team the next night. But my messages weren't complicated—they were simply to think positively, support team camaraderie, work hard, and be persistent. All four are important, but the first two in particular directly address girls' needs.

BFFS VERSUS BUDDIES IN ARMS

The nature of girls is quite different from that of boys. My term for groups of boys is "buddies in arms." Whereas girl athletes tend toward best friendship and collaborative, emotional relationships, boy athletes line up in order of dominance in teams and have activity-based, cognitive (thinking) relationships. With teenage girls in particular, you will often hear them talking on and on about their relationships in an emotional manner. Not so with the buddies-in-arms style of boy athletes. In fact, boys generally don't understand what makes girls talk about and stay so focused on relationships, especially with their boyfriends and friends in high school. The generally more cooperative nature of girls helps them to show more openness to new ideas simply because they want to please others; on the other hand, girls can be tough on each other and struggle to deal with rivalries with peers during their teenage years. Many coaches and players think it's more important for girls to get along with their teammates on a personal level than it is for boys—which leads to the BFFs thesis. Boys look more at ability than anything when they play on teams together. They play to compete and win, not necessarily to be friends. And boys seem to have a much easier time competing with each other and then stepping away from the game as friends.

In my research for this book, I was fortunate enough to have the opportunity to interview two young women who play high school softball and are best friends. Becca and Aria have been constant companions in softball since third grade, and now they play on a high school and club team together. Even their mothers are best friends and partners in a business. Becca describes herself as outgoing, focused, determined to be better, and overly supportive at times. Aria sees herself as hardworking, persistent, and detail oriented. Both of them have the same motto: "Strive for the best in yourself." Becca commented, "Aria helps when I'm mentally not there and I feel comfortable with her telling me when I totally mess up." Aria talks about her relationship with Becca in the following way: "Our friendship is good fun. We pick each other up when we're down. She's my other half and my biggest competition."

These girls both have significant family support. In eighth grade, Becca was feeling down and wanting to quit softball—so her entire extended family got together and played a fun game of softball, which improved Becca's attitude about the game and made her want to keep playing. Aria is a star player—she won the MCAL (the North Coast Section of the California Interscholastic Federation) triple crown (she had the highest batting average, most home runs, and highest runs batted in) in her sophomore year of high school—and is also apparently the more outgoing of the two girls. She was recruited for a softball scholarship as a young freshman and has a scholarship to Loyola Marymount University beginning in fall of 2014. Becca, who is a year younger, is still waiting to find the right school. Notably, unlike female athletes of the past, these teens have a wide array of role models to look up to and university scholarships to choose from, as well as one another to depend on for support. When I asked them how much of their self-esteem is tied to sports, they both responded, "All of it"—and Aria very astutely labeled sports as their way of performing, the means by which they get positive attention.

The main exception to the rule that girls in sports have BFFs who support them primarily occurs when girls are raised mainly around brothers and by fathers or when their sporting activities tend toward more independent styles. Marla Streb, for example, a retired professional downhill mountain biker and recent inductee into the US Mountain Bike Hall of Fame, was raised with four rough-and-tumble brothers. While growing up with them, she first engaged in her risk-taking sports behavior, including quarry jumping and off-road go-carting. She had to work hard to keep up with her brothers, which taught her to persist and never give up or whine. And she continued to play sports as a teen, which provided her with a way to express herself and bond with her brothers. Her closest brother, Mark, encouraged her to push the envelope, enjoy the outdoors, and love life and live it to the fullest. She didn't have a female BFF—but she did have a strong support system and a brother who was her BFF. Unfortunately, Mark unexpectedly died while serving in the Peace Corps when Marla was only eighteen years old. She was understandably devastated and got into some self-destructive behavior for a while. Marla did recover and continued in the fun, risky sports behavior that Mark had encouraged her to participate in while he was alive.

COMPETITION AND TEENAGE GIRLS AND BOYS

In the area where I live, there is intense focus on girls playing and competing in sports. In fact, high numbers of girls from the Bay Area start playing sports at a young age and end up with college scholarships. These girls learn to play competitive sports early on, and as they enter puberty, they become even more comfortable with competition. Much insecurity can pop up for girls and boys alike during the teen years. Sports often help girls deal better with these insecurities, but they don't necessarily help them deal better with competition. With girls' need to collaborate and feel valued, overcoming their aversion to competition, even in sports, can prove a daunting task.

In a research study from the Melpomene Institute in Minnesota, an organization that strives to empower girls and women to achieve full, healthy lives, researchers compared soccer-playing girls' and boys' attitudes toward competition. The study was heavily loaded with girls (557 to only 320 boys); the subjects were mainly white (84 percent), were between the ages of twelve and seventeen, and were primarily high academic achievers (in the eighty-first percentile). The researchers discovered striking differences in how the sexes viewed aspects of competition. When asked to respond to the statement "I would do almost anything to win," only 29 percent of the girls marked the most affirmative choice, "frequently and almost always." Of the boys, meanwhile, 49 percent answered the same statement affirmatively. In response to the second statement, "It is more important for key players to play in order to win than for everyone to get equal playing time," only 24 percent of the girls (but 42 percent of the boys) responded "frequently and almost always." Finally, in response to the statement "I get very upset when my team loses," 18 percent of the girls and 42 percent of the boys chose the most affirmative answer.[8]

So it seems that boys and girls view competition in different ways— but what does all this mean? The data may suggest that girls are not willing to do just anything to win and that they wish to be inclusive and may feel the need to win within the guidelines of fair play and avoiding conflict. These inferences are drawn from the strengths of the female brain that Dr. Daniel Amen highlights in his research. Teenage girls are relational by nature, which gives rise to a fair amount of inclusiveness and not wanting to leave their teammates out, which certainly affects their approach to competition. There are also those "mean girls" mentioned earlier, who purposely leave other girls out as they sort out where they belong in the typical high school groups, but they are not typical of the general female population. Teenage girls need to learn what I call "female collaborative competition," involving hard work, collaboration with each other, and of course, having fun while competing.

Lindsay Gottlieb, head coach of Cal Berkeley's girls' basketball team, spoke of the importance of getting to know her players so that when she had to make the hard decisions about who would stay on the bench, her players would regard it as a team decision rather than a personal one. Teenage girls need to learn this lesson as a foundation principle in order to prepare for the collegiate level of competition. Donna de Varona, a cofounder of the Women's Sports Foundation, labels this fair play ideal as the "right value of sport."

TEENS' BIOLOGY

The increasing estrogen in girls during the teen years adds to their feeling and recalling the emotion of stressful events like sports competitions. They remember what happens in more emotional detail and for longer periods than boys. The female brain has strong connectors between both the right and left hemispheres, with language and emotion centers in each one. This may lead to increased sensitivity in girls about the outcomes of their sports competitions, both during high school and when they become adults. In contrast, the rising level of testosterone in boys contributes to their greater levels of aggression and stronger physical development. This biological difference means that the goal of spoken communication with female teens must be to encourage and push them toward playing their best. Male teens tend to brush off harsh or sarcastic words and often joke with the peers they compete with before, during, and after games, but girls take negative words and competition more to heart.

Teenage girls depend on their sporting circles, and especially their best friends, to support them in their sports pursuits throughout high school. Athletic teens need other athletic teen friendships to help them remain in sports and not feel isolated in doing so. Positive relationships are key to girls enjoying sports and playing their best. Becca and Aria, the teenage softball players we met earlier in this chapter, illustrate the strength and positive impact of sports-centered friendships in young girls' lives.

GIRLS' AND WOMEN'S EMPOWERMENT THROUGH SPORTS

The Women's Sports Foundation was created in 1974 to improve and grow the sporting lives of girls and women. It has said from the beginning that girls and women need strong support systems—in fact, the organization's first president, Donna de Varona, said that relationships are the whole issue for women athletes. Years ago, long before much of the research we have access to today had been conducted, this association recognized girls' need to collaborate, bond, and have best friends.

In 2012, Hillary Clinton led the US Department of State in its Empowering Women and Girls through Sports Initiative, the main goal of which is to empower girls and develop female athletes all over the world. For the first time, the government is actively encouraging girls to set up networks and reach out to other athletes in a more global way. And this kind of networking begins at a young age, as collaboration and connection are essential for girls to lead full, healthy lives and for them to learn leadership, loyalty, and ultimately friendship. The initiative's ultimate goal is to encourage girls' and women's involvement in leadership in schools, in the workplace, and in society as a whole. Its committee is made up of many high-powered former female athletes, including Donna de Varona (who, in addition to serving as president of the Women's Sports Foundation, set a world record in swimming the individual medley at age thirteen in 1960), and Julie Foudy and Mia Hamm (both members of the 1996 Olympic gold-medal-winning women's soccer team and the "Fab Five" of soccer). Ultimately, the organization provides a broader vision for girls, allowing them to look outward and realize that sports can help all female athletes to reach across the table to others. Speaking to the importance of the concept of best friends forever, this initiative is focused on encouraging and developing friendships between teen, collegiate, and pro female athletes from around the world.

TEN MENTAL STRATEGIES FOR TEENAGE BFFS

1. Make girlfriends who are athletic like you.
2. Find girlfriends to train and work out with.
3. Listen to your friends, and talk to them as well.
4. Encourage yourself and your BFF to think positively about sports.
5. Learn to set up athletic goals and objectives and discuss them with a girlfriend.
6. Speak up for your girlfriends. Have their backs.
7. Strive for your mentors to become your friends.

8. Learn to be friendly with your competitors.
9. Participate in social activities outside of sports with your BFFs.
10. Remember, we all need each other. Have compassion for those who are suffering and struggling to fit in.

3

THE FAMILY THAT PLAYS TOGETHER STAYS TOGETHER

If there's one thing I've learned in my years as a sports psychologist, it's that female athletes are most successful when they have the help of a supportive family. Girls with parents who support all of their children's respective athletic pursuits—who teach them to appreciate challenges and to strive to do the best that they can do rather than focus solely on outcomes—excel in sports. We see this in recent (and not-so-recent) Olympics, where various teams have included siblings.

For female athletes, attitude is key, but in the United States we focus way too much on results and not enough on the value of simply participating in sports. It's crucial to reframe this perspective—to teach girls that regardless of the outcome, the real reward of sports lies in working hard to improve personal performance. And mothers are often the parents who understand this. In fact, it's usually mothers, not fathers, who bring their daughters in to see me or to attend my workshops. They tend to be the key family members to connect with what their daughters need in order to thrive as athletes. But everyone has a role to play: fathers need to learn to communicate with their daughters in an effective way, and siblings who support each other in sports help round out a healthy family system. At the end of the day, the family with a true love and passion for sports is the one that girls and women will thrive in as athletes.

POSITIVE VERSUS NEGATIVE FAMILY INFLUENCES

When families devote the bulk of their time and energy to their children's athletic endeavors, this can lead to both positive and negative consequences. On the one hand, athletes who receive strong family support tend to thrive—in fact, most of the women I interviewed for this book (including Olympian, pro, and amateur athletes) report having positive family relationships, particularly regarding their sports lives, and they credit their families with helping them to pursue and succeed in the sports they love. On the other hand, problems can arise within a family when parents are overly invested in the athletic success of their children—if they push too hard, for example, for their child to be the best. And parents' involvement is important for both boys and girls when it comes to sports, but research suggests that a family's role is actually "more important for girls' athletic involvement than for boys' involvement."[1]

Support for girls and women athletes is best delivered by talking in a reasonable voice. Yelling, taking a loud, harsh, critical tone, and giving nonspecific instructions usually causes females to underperform. Some do succeed despite this, but sports then becomes a punitive and not fun activity. This is especially true in middle and high school. Parents need to take heed that excessive pressure and negativity contribute to poor results and take away the fun quotient that is so important to girls and women in sports. A certain amount of support from parents is vital to girls feeling positive about their competitive sporting experiences.

Julia Mancuso, the Olympic skier we met in chapter 1, had a tight-knit sports family growing up. She was surrounded by strong female athletic role models: her grandmother started Gym Marin in 1973 (a gym focused solely on gymnastics); her aunt Lucia, the first woman in the family to benefit from the passage of Title IX, was Stanford's first female gymnast; and many others in her immediate and extended family of aunts and female cousins are athletic. When I asked her about what she thought helped her become such a successful athlete, Julia responded, "Just growing up with such strong females surrounding me, I always had a good self-image and outgoing personality. . . . My parents have always been very athletic. Every family vacation always revolved around some sort of sport." Her aunt Lucia, meanwhile, describes a tiara Julia received from her coach in 2005 as a "symbol of our family, having a lot of heart, a lot of love" and as a community where "you don't have to worry about judgments."

Katheryn Curi Mattis, a former Webcor pro cyclist, enjoyed the encouragement of an athletically oriented family growing up as well. According to Katheryn, all the "Curi kids were jocks," and her parents were "unbelievably supportive." Her father encouraged Katheryn, her two sisters, and her brother, as kids, to participate in a Sunday activity at their home that Katheryn dubbed the "Wide World of Sports Sunday"—a sort of obstacle course that involved swimming laps in their pool, running around the house a designated number of times, and finishing off with shooting a series of short layups. And Katheryn and all of her siblings were sent to a private school that treated sports as a significant part of the curriculum. They all learned to compete and have fun together. Katheryn says her dad's motto was, "If you're really passionate about something, do it."

When a family invests too much in an athlete's endeavors, of course, it can have an adverse effect on everyone involved. I worked with one young female dancer, for example, who suddenly decided she wanted to stop dancing and change her lifestyle—right as she was in the middle of auditioning for professional troupes. The family had organized their entire lives and their whole identity around her development as a professional dancer, and the idea that she might abandon everything they had worked for was a crushing blow to all of them. She was not to be swayed, however; she felt guilty for letting everyone down but was quite clear in her decision. Her family members had a long, hard road ahead in terms of working through their disappointment.

On the other end of the spectrum is Lisa Lopez, an all-American miler from the University of California, Berkeley. Lisa's father played on the national Nicaraguan baseball team, so he was an athlete in his own right, but he just couldn't seem to accept, support, or encourage Lisa in her own athletic pursuits. He was very controlling and did not approve of her running. "He was afraid I was going to end up barefoot and pregnant," Lisa told me. Luckily for Lisa, her mother and two brothers (who ran cross-country and track) were supportive of her, and she kept running. She eventually received a full cross-country scholarship to University of California, Berkeley, transferring from the City College of San Francisco and even went on to become captain of her team. She hails her mother as her pillar and as the parent who saw "the light at the end of the tunnel" regarding her running.

Like Lisa, I had parents who conveyed mixed messages about sports, especially prior to the passage of Title IX in 1972. Both of my parents were tall, serious, and athletic—but my mother was always embarrassed by her 5′9″ stature (which was especially tall for a woman of her generation), and she was uncomfortable with the fact that I was a tomboy. When I won a spot on my high school's first cross-country team, my mother insisted that running was not ladylike enough and refused to give me permission to join.

My father, in contrast, treated me like a son when it came to sports. From a very young age, I learned from him how to swim, dive, golf, ride horses, backpack, canoe, and play tennis and badminton. From ages ten to twelve, I played badminton as his doubles partner on the indoor court at Oswego Lake Country Club; yet golf remained the primary sport for my mother and father. As with all sports, these badminton matches were a serious affair. My father's intensity and competitiveness often took the fun out of things. Yet, I was such a good badminton player that my dad expressed few complaints. These games were the happiest times playing sports with him that I remember. In juxtaposition, my mother wanted me to be a lady. In her eyes, tennis and badminton were permissible as lady's sports, but that didn't mean she supported my involvement in either one—in fact, neither of my parents ever attended any of my sports tournaments. My mother even went so far as to send me to charm school in an attempt to make me less of a tomboy (it didn't work). She remained ambivalent about her daughter (and herself) competing in sports. In my early twenties, she changed her tune as I began participating in running events at age twenty-four.

WORKING TOGETHER AS A FAMILY

An Olympic silver medalist in basketball in 1986 and one of the top ten female athletes of the twentieth century according to *Time* magazine, Ann Meyers Drysdale is a shining example of a female from a family of multiple athletes with total support for everyone. All ten of her siblings participated in sports, including basketball, track, football, baseball, swimming, tennis, and softball. Ann herself played seven sports in high school—track, basketball, tennis, volleyball, field hockey, softball, and badminton—which was extraordinary for a girl athlete at that time. In fact, Ann and I played on the badminton and tennis teams together. Her father of Polish and German descent played basketball in 1945 for Marquette University in Wisconsin. Sports participation was a given in Ann's large Catholic family. Although Ann's accomplishments are vast and varied, her older brother, Dave, played pro ball for the Milwaukee Bucks. She describes her younger sister, Patty, as the best athlete of them all. Patty played softball for California State University, Fullerton, and pro softball in Florida. Ann expresses deep respect and admiration for her sister, and she made it sound like her family members all bonded with each other around their respective sports. "We all supported each other by attending and cheering at each other's games. Mom was the biggest cheerleader for all of us!"

The influence of the family for Ann taught her to compete with respect and fun. Her parents emphasized "chores done and education first," then sports second. During her teen years, Ann was impacted by lots of people. She focused on the lessons her parents were teaching all the kids. Her parents emphasized a "strong work ethic." Whatever you do, work hard, and be committed. Be "determined" to set goals and accomplish them. Be "dedicated" since the "feeling brings you back for more." All eleven of the kids enjoyed playing sports. "We played for the love of it."

THE IMPORTANCE OF THE MOTHER-DAUGHTER RELATIONSHIP

The mother-daughter relationship is one of the most important in a girl's athletic life. Dads do play a significant role (especially single fathers, of course), but for most girls, their moms play the key role. In a 2008 Women's Sports Foundation study, in fact, girl athletes ranked their mothers as number one for supporting them in sports. From a professional standpoint, I can say that I have watched many moms interact with their daughters over the years, and I have seen how the mother-daughter relationship can make or break a young woman's involvement in competitive sports. Without maternal support, or if there is an underlying maternal conflict, girls' sports performance often suffers. Because of this, it's important that, whether or not they have been athletes, mothers of female athletes play a supportive role for their daughters. When you attend meets, games, races, and performances, listen to the best way you can assist your daughter. Do not expect her to take care of your emotional needs and any anxiety you experience from her competition in sports.

Research suggests that previously or currently athletic mothers are more likely than nonathletic mothers to encourage their daughters to participate in sports, and they are better equipped to support their daughters' efforts. Christine Thorburn, a 2004 and 2008 Olympic road cyclist and physician, is a living example of this trend. She grew up on seven acres in Iowa in an athletic household where everybody did some type of sport. Her mother often took Christine and her siblings to sporting events, including cross-country, track, and bike races, teaching them early on to enjoy the spirit of competition.

One story Christine told me stood out as particularly representative of how parents affect their children's attitude toward sports. She was in kindergarten, and the whole family was riding bikes to a community picnic and parade. It was a seven-mile ride, and on the way to the picnic, five-year-old Christine was having trouble keeping up with the family. After the parade, her mom and dad wanted to put her in a friend's car for the return home, but Christine refused and promised to keep up on the way home. Her mom good-naturedly agreed, and Christine fulfilled her promised—in fact, she rode so hard that she ended up way ahead of her mom. "My mother gave me room to do what I wanted, which allowed me to constantly set goals and meet them," Christine explains. Today, she describes herself as competitive, stubborn, and focused, and she credits her mother with helping to cultivate those traits.

Stacey Johnson, a former 1980 Olympic fencer, had the opposite experience from Christine: her mom just didn't know what to make of her daughter's involvement in sports. Stacey's mother often made negative comments about her enjoyment of sports and encouraged her to quit. In fact, Stacey told me, at one point her mother outright exclaimed, "When are you going to move on from sports?" Shannon Hartnett, a three-time world champion in powerlifting, had a mother who only "tolerated" sports. Her parents fought all the time, however, so sports became Shannon's escape from chaos. For her, "being able to control one thing provided a focus and released my energy." Clearly, both of these women succeeded in their sport of choice even without the support of their parents. Based on my observations, however, they are not representative of the majority but exceptions to the rule.

In the work that I've done over the years, I've developed a model for the five most common types of moms of teenage girl athletes:

1. Assertive, analytical, and supportive
2. Supportive and encouraging
3. Passive and pleasing
4. Aggressive and pressuring
5. Absent and removed

The first type, the analytical and supportive type of mom, knows everything about and is actively involved with her daughter's sporting life. Athletic moms tend to be grouped in this category. Of the athletes I've worked with, one mother in particular belonged to this type. Darcy, a teenage softball player, was having trouble on the mound; she had a difficult time handling her frustration, and a couple of bad pitches could ruin an entire game for her. Her mom, Karen, initiated contact with me, and though initially hesitant, Darcy got into the swing of things right away. I decided to try including her mother in the process, and Darcy seemed to enjoy her mom's involvement. From then on, I saw her alone for the first forty-five or so minutes, then brought her mom in for the last fifteen minutes. Both mother and daughter appeared to benefit from this type of working together, and Darcy eventually learned how to deal effectively with her frustration and got accepted to the college of her choice on a softball scholarship.

The second type of mother, the supportive and encouraging type, is different from the first type in that, although she might take her daughter to and from training and go to her meets, she does not ask many questions and may have difficulty understanding the technical aspects of her daughter's sport(s). This type generally tends to be the mom who never really played sports and isn't interested in or doesn't understand the details of how they work. In working with a young swimmer, I encountered an unusual situation with her mother. Her mother suffered an illness that left her short- and long-term memory damaged. She showed great interest in her daughter's athletics but couldn't remember facts about them or her daughter's appointments. She often called me to ask when the appointments were scheduled. This was difficult for her daughter to accept. The mother tried to support and encourage her daughter in sports but had physical restrictions. The problem became the fact that her daughter was not able or willing to accept her mother's limitations and inabilities.

The third type of mother, the passive and pleasing type, lets her daughter take the lead and does everything she can to help her. I once dealt with a teenage dancer whose mom brought her to me for help with her confidence. We worked on building her daughter's confidence for a number of months using such techniques as recalling past successful performances and practicing positive thoughts, and ultimately she achieved a more solid sense of confidence in her performing and sense of self in general. At the end of our work together, however, she relayed to her mom that she wasn't as interested in dancing as she once had been and told her that she wanted to reduce her involvement. This totally confused her mom. Her mom assumed everything was fine with continuing to dance, but it became clear that the lack of communication between them about her daughter's lack of desire, despite her talent, differed from her mom's expectations.

The fourth type of mother, the aggressive and pressuring type, causes undue stress related to her daughter's performance in sports. She's the one getting in the coach's face, overestimating her daughter's skills, and holding her out as "special"; she's the one placing extra pressure on her daughter to perform and accomplish goals that may actually be her own. This type of mom is the one most likely to push her daughter so hard that she either embarrasses her or pushes her out of sports altogether. Years ago, I worked with a young swimmer, Lucy, who was filled with anxiety and was highly self-critical. Initially she portrayed her mother as someone who kept everything under control but was relatively relaxed—but after working with her for a while, I realized how aggressive her mother's behavior truly was and how she was constantly pressuring Lucy to do better. Through our work together, despite Lucy's using the key words and phrases of "confident," "prepared," "relaxed," and "enjoying myself," Lucy's mother seemed to pressure her more, causing her to get more frustrated than ever. Although Lucy got better at not coming down too hard on herself after races, her mother's attitude seemed to undermine her improvement. In another instance, a mom brought her fifteen-year-old daughter, Lilly, a cross-country runner, to push her to perform better. They were having problems with the school team because the mom wouldn't even encourage or allow Lilly to work out with her teammates.

The coach became insistent about Lilly joining the team for workouts. It soon became clear that the mom was driving her daughter away from her teammates and other girlfriends. The mom was totally focused on what she wanted for her daughter without truly considering her daughter's needs.

The fifth and last type, the absent and removed mother, is harmful to her daughter's sporting life through her neglect and noninvolvement. Particularly during their teenage years, girls need a certain amount of involvement and support from their moms, and mothers who are not present often make their daughters feel forgotten, unimportant, and neglected. One teenage basketball player I worked with, Audrey, had a mother so uninterested in her sport participation that the idea of her mother attending games hadn't even occurred to her. Audrey also didn't seem to understand her teammates' interest in "girly" activities like clothes shopping and getting mani-pedis and thought they were a waste of time. She wanted to spend all her time practicing and not having much fun. Her apparent lack of desire to bond with her basketball teammates was unusual for a teenage girl of her age. Moms' participation in her girl teens' life and upbringing is essential for teenage girls to feel loved and exposed to their feminine nature. Audrey came to see me because her father yelled too much at her games, and once her dad greatly reduced that behavior, Audrey felt our work was done. Throughout our sessions, her mom remained uninvolved, and I couldn't help but see how that affected Audrey's performance and attitude toward her sport and other girls.

ADVICE TO MOTHERS: SUPPORTING YOUR ATHLETIC DAUGHTER

Girls who participate in sports are less likely to drop out of school and more likely to attend and graduate from college and obtain good jobs. Participating in sports promotes self-esteem, discipline, and confidence, and it's fun, too—a benefit that shouldn't be underestimated. Girls' minds are drawn to collaborating and bonding with others and giving and receiving positive feedback. When they have good role models and constructive support, these are things that sports can offer them. As a mother, you can support your athletic daughter by doing the following:

- Suggesting she find other female athletes to hold up as role models
- Providing opportunities for her to meet and spend time with other female athletes
- Allowing her to take risks
- Helping her learn how to manage her sports-related stress
- Talking with her about your own sports experiences, if you are or were an athlete
- Letting her develop her own pre-event routine
- Attending her meets, games, or races

FATHERS AS MENTORS

For many girls and women, fathers may still remain the predominant role model, especially when it comes to sports. Mothers may be the family members most likely to support and encourage their daughters, but fathers are often the parent with a better understanding of sports because a greater number of them have direct athletic experiences of their own. But the main difference between mothers and fathers lies in their brain chemistry: unlike women, men generally bond around activities, view relationships in a cognitive manner, and feel uncomfortable talking with their daughters about feelings. Traditionally, feelings discussions are the domain of mothers.

A study in the *Journal of Human Communication*[2] looked at forty-three adult females (aged twenty-two and up) and forty-three fathers (aged forty-five to seventy) to explore the importance of the father-daughter relationship and the different communication styles between fathers and daughters. The researchers found that sports were the most frequently identified activity that helped fathers and daughters bond. Peggy Drexler, one of the study's authors, has asserted that passage of Title IX in 1972 played a big role in this as implementation of that law opened up a whole world of opportunities to girls and women, especially in sports. "Sports became a great bridge to draw girls into activities with their fathers," Drexler said, and "a strong relationship between father and daughter can set up a girl for success later in life."[3]

Julia Violich, a forty-seven-year-old competitive mountain biker and Bear Development racing team coach, says her father was the primary parent to support her athletic pursuits. Having played water polo and swum competitively at Stanford, he encouraged her to get involved with sports throughout her life. Her parents separated when she was eight, creating a difficult emotional time for Julia. But, as always, she rallied and went at sports with a vengeance. As a younger girl and teenager, she primarily played soccer. She was the athlete, not her brother. She became captain of at her high school team, and while she was still in school, her dad started the first select soccer league in Marin County, California, where they lived. In college, Julia switched to mountain biking as her primary sport of choice, and her dad continued to offer his unwavering support. Today Julia remains a strong, persistent, hardworking athlete—and her dad is part of the reason why.

Professional Women's National Basketball Association player Natalie Williams gives her father, Nate Williams—who played in the National Basketball Association for a number of years with a variety of teams—a lot of credit for supporting her basketball career. She has many accolades, including being the first woman to earn all-American honors in both basketball and volleyball and being named "Female Athlete of the Century" by her home state, Utah. She believes that she's inherited her father's power and strength.

Perhaps surprisingly, research shows that girls raised by single fathers are just as well adjusted as those raised by single mothers. Fathers appear to have the most significant impact on their daughters in sports, academics, and careers. Girls learn through sports such habits as discipline, commitment, and structure. With a good father, they learn the importance of respect for authority. "A daughter has a better relationship with her father when her mother does not rely on her for advice or comfort on adult issues—especially issues involving the parents' relationship with each other."[4]

ADVICE TO FATHERS: SUPPORTING YOUR ATHLETIC DAUGHTER

The biggest piece of advice that I can give fathers in supporting their daughters as athletes is to talk and listen to them about more than just the technicalities of their sport. Unlike for boys, sports will always have an emotional component for girls. If they cry, just let them. Don't try to fix the situation. They will express feelings with positive and negative results. Their expression about sports will differ from your sons'. Female athletes thrive on support from their relationships and generally respond poorly to being pushed too hard or screamed at. (As discussed in chapter 1, even women at high levels of athleticism get turned off by aggressive screaming.) That said, as a father, you can support your athletic daughter by doing the following:

- Talking and listening to her about her specific sport and life
- Being supportive and not highly confrontational, even when critiquing her performance
- Letting her set her own athletic goals unless she asks for help
- Helping her to focus on personal bests and not just on competition.
- Focusing on keeping sports fun
- Letting her live her own dreams and not trying to impose yours upon her
- Allowing her to develop her own pre-event routines
- Attending her meets, games, or races

SIBLINGS AS ALLIES AND COMPETITORS

A recent study of siblings that looked at birth order, sibling sport participation, and sports expertise development discovered that top-level athletes were more likely to be later-born siblings.[5] The study's authors concluded that older siblings often help their younger siblings learn to participate in sports, which means that having siblings as allies in sports may have a significant effect upon subsequent athletic success.[6]

When it comes to girls in sports, however, sibling rivalry can be either helpful or harmful. When female siblings compete in sports together, either on a team or individually, some form of rivalry will exist. This can be a positive experience, but if the parents handle it poorly, or if the siblings don't get along in general, it can be just the opposite. Our female nature (our brain and socialization) includes a desire to bond, collaborate, and empathize. Research has pinpointed these qualities through the use of brain scans. A new study published in the journal *Pediatrics*[7] suggests that when it entails more than just friendly competition, aggression between siblings can cause real psychological trauma. One sibling can also feel neglected or become jealous if the other is a more successful athlete and gets an inordinate amount of attention as a result. These kinds of tensions can turn into grudges that sometimes carry on into adulthood. Teaching siblings, especially girls, to deal with competition in a healthy way, however, can help them learn to cooperate, collaborate, manage frustration, and effectively handle problems or conflicts. [8]

Honor Fetherston, a top Masters runner during the 1990s, is an identical triplet who grew up sharing her love of running with her two sisters, Shelley and Sharon. Their father was an air force general, and they moved around a lot—but instead of causing discord within the family, this only served to create a tighter bond between Honor and her sisters. Together, they ran at significantly competitive levels during high school; together, they all qualified for state championships in Washington State. The sisters were often seen chasing each other around the track. They share everything and are best friends. All three qualified and ran the hundredth Boston Marathon together. They are all supportive of one another in sports and life. And when in 1994, at age forty, Honor set and held the Masters half-marathon record at the Las Vegas Half and then qualified for the Olympic trials, both of her sisters were ecstatic about her accomplishments. Shelley and Sharon showed a lot of "excitement and support when I was a competitive Masters level runner," Honor said. "They were behind me the whole way." She told me that her top reason for participating in sports is to have fun, the motivation that she and her sisters always shared as triplets.

Earlier, I spoke about the athletic closeness of Christine Thorburn's tight-knit athletic family. There was camaraderie around sports with siblings and parents. Christine became a runner. She felt like she had to run to be close to her dad, who was a distance runner. Christine looked up to her sister and respected her as she provided a role model for her running and her competitive nature. She eventually switched to cycling, in which she excelled and became an Olympian. Even though Christine considered herself, in retrospect, the annoying, bratty little sister, her older sister expressed pride in Christine's accomplishments.

Erin Maxwell, a world-class 4.7 sailor, learned to sail alongside her two younger brothers. Her dad, the athletic parent, participated actively in sailing and running. He encouraged Erin and her two younger brothers to learn how to sail, and she began taking sailing classes at the age of six, eventually, having lessons in the morning and the evening. Erin and her brothers all took to sailing. Their involvement developed a bond among them. Her dad pushed them to take competition seriously and to enjoy applying strategy and tactics. Over the years, Erin competed head-to-head with her brother J.R., a friendly competition that consistently challenged both of them to improve. Today, Erin's brothers still sail competitively as well, but Erin is the star. In 2008, she and her partner, Isabelle Kinsolving, won the 470 (small, two-person sailboat) World Championships in Melbourne, Australia, with her family's blessing and support. Erin is quick to note that her family directly shaped her athletic development.

Taylor and Connie Ellett are a remarkable pair of young sisters who compete together on the Northern Illinois University (NIU) golf team. Both of their parents were college players—in fact, their mother, Sue, was a pioneering member of NIU's first women's golf team in 1986. With two golfers as parents, the girls learned how to play at an early age—Taylor at seven, Connie at six. Growing up as golfers has provided the sisters a unique opportunity to support each other in sport. They drive each other to improve. "We both push each other to be better," Taylor said of her sister in one interview. "We both have very different personalities, but we balance each other out as far as combativeness goes. We work really well together, and it's been a great experience to have her as a teammate and as a sister." These female siblings are a great illustration of the idea of collaborative competition, each supporting the other and wanting her to play her best. [9]

Olympic Siblings

Taking a moment to look back at past US Olympic teams, we can find a number of wonderful role models that exemplify healthy sister-sister and sister-brother competitive duos. Multiple pairs of siblings competed in the 2012 London Olympics for Team USA. In fact, the 2012 Olympics had more females (269) than males (261) for the first time ever. There were also a number of siblings competing, including both sister-sister and brother-sister combinations. The best known, of course, are the Williams sisters, who have competed together in tennis doubles in three Olympic Games and received gold medals every time. They seem to have established a good working relationship, particularly in their doubles play, and they also support one another by watching each other's matches. Despite the pressure of the high-level competition they participate in, they have managed to remain friends.

Two other sisters who competed in the London Olympics were Alyssa and Haley Anderson, both swimmers and Olympic medalists. Haley, in particular, is known for her smiling, happy, positive demeanor, and their family is very supportive. In fact, before her Olympic race, Haley was smiling, talking, and having fun. Her mother expresses how proud the whole family is of both sisters. Haley won a silver medal in the 10K open-water swim, and Alyssa won a gold medal in the 4 × 200 freestyle relay. Both experienced a bunch of encouragement from family, with parents, sisters, and aunts attending their Olympic events. Many family members and extended relatives came to cheer them on in 2012. The sisters used their allotted twelve tickets to cover the large family contingent in the stands at both the start and the finish.[i]

Julia and Katie Reinprecht, who competed together on the 2012 Olympic field hockey team and also played together on the Princeton Tigers field hockey team, took the year off from school, moved to California, and trained hard with their team before the London games. They both say that training together created a closer bond between them.

Among the best-known Olympic brother-sister competitors are Jackie Joyner-Kersee and Al Joyner, both gold medalists in Olympic track and field. Jackie and Al grew up in a poor area of East St.

Louis, across from a liquor store and pool hall in a neighborhood with periodic shootings (in fact, Jackie saw a man get shot right in front of her house when she was only eleven years old). Both siblings vowed to make it out via sports, and they succeeded: Jackie attended the University of California, Los Angeles, where she competed in both track and field and basketball, and Al attended Arkansas State University, where he competed in the triple jump in track and field. In 1984, both qualified for and competed in the Olympic Games in Los Angeles. The rest is history. Al received an Olympic gold medal for the triple jump, the first won by an American in eighty years. Jackie, the younger sister, became a four-time Olympian. In heptathlon, she received a silver medal in 1988 and a gold medal in 1998 and 1992. In long jump, she received a gold medal in 1988 and two bronze medals in 1992 and 1996. *Sports Illustrated* later named her "Greatest Female Athlete of the 20th Century." Jackie has long said that her brother's support, encouragement, and advice made a critical difference in her life. To this day, they remain close friends, siblings-in-arms, and, perhaps most importantly, excellent role models for other brother-sister athletes.

[i] Deirdre Fitzpatrick, "Team USA Sisters Compete in Olympic Swimming," WXII12.com, August 7, 2012, http://www.wxii12.com/sports/2014-olympics/Team-USA-sisters-compete-in-Olympic-swimming/16005138.

HOW PARENTS SUPPORT HEALTHY COMPETITION BETWEEN FEMALE ATHLETES AND THEIR SIBLINGS

A female athlete's siblings are always going to play a role in her life—and some level of rivalry is natural. It is parents' responsibility to teach children how to handle competition with their siblings and ensure that any rivalry doesn't become excessive or unhealthy. Research suggests that focusing on building positive relationships between siblings is the best way to handle this rivalry. Listen to your daughter's feelings. If she feels left out or neglected in her sports, you need to examine your behavior toward her. When there are two sibling athletes, never pit them against each in an aggressive manner. This is especially true for female siblings because encouraging such aggression sets them up to be overly competitive, which can lead to resentment and dislike from other athletes, as well as insecurity within themselves. Conversely, if girl siblings learn to compete with one another in a friendly, fun way, they can help and push each other to succeed.

FAMILY DYNAMICS AND FEMALE ATHLETES

Research has often illustrated that family dynamics directly influence how female athletes approach their sport(s). Overly high and overly low expectations from a young female athlete's family, especially her parents, are directly associated with reduced interest in sports. Girls with family members who participate in, enjoy, and commit to sports without being too pushy, however, are much more likely to succeed as they get older. For parents, this means being present and invested without being overly critical. After a disappointing sports event, when providing advice, parents should try to start with mentioning one positive prior to saying anything negative. Girls take feedback much more personally than boys and are more likely to internalize sports-related critiques as criticisms of themselves and their value as a person.

Support and encouragement from the family are essential for all female athletes, even elite performers. Kami Semick, a top US ultrarunner, told me that her husband and daughter frequently travel with her to her races, and they participate by volunteering for the race in some way. Kami sees it as a mutually beneficial practice for her and her family—she receives the support she needs, and she gets to provide her daughter with a positive and inspiring role model.

Talking, collaboration, and bonding are the three most powerful pulls in a woman's brain—that's why girls and women generally feel better about competing in races, events, games, and meets when they have their family's support. With family or friends present, they are more likely to perform well as long as no one yells critically. Be encouraging. Be a cheerleader. There's nothing more a woman wants to see at the end of a race. I've experienced this myself on multiple occasions. Several years ago, for example, I was running a 50K, and my husband and our two perpetually happy golden retrievers, Spencer and Parker, came to "crew" for me. Throughout the race, the three of them showed up at each aid station to cheer me on, and just knowing they were there made the time and the race go by faster. It was my first 50K in fourteen years, but I finished it with no problem, largely because I knew that JP and the dogs would be there waiting for me at the finish line. It didn't just feel good to know that I was loved and supported by my family—it made me keep going until the finish.

In the sport of ultrarunning (running more than 26.2 miles), crews are critical in providing support, good cheer, physical needs, special foods, and even help with pacing. Sometimes if you don't have family support, you build your own family through the sports that you're in. In 1992, when I ran my first hundred-mile-mile race (Vermont 100), I went alone without crew, pacer, or family. At that time, I wasn't very good at asking people for support. A number of my friends (all men at that time) were running the race, so some of their crew (mostly women) had offered to help out, but only if their partners and I were similarly paced. Occasionally, this worked out. However, I had worked on training every part of my body, so I was in great shape and happy at every rest stop. An interesting event occurred. The local guy recruited to pace me was nowhere to be found at the pacer pickup point at mile seventy, but California ultrarunning legend John Medinger showed up instead. "Tropical John," as he's now called, popped up out of the night and explained that he had never seen a one-hundred-mile runner in such a good mood throughout the race. John usually only paced fast guys, and the runner he was supposed to pace had dropped out. He told me that he was going to pace me since I appeared so happy. What a relief to have John, an experienced ultrarunner, pacing me. He set up goals for me and told me what to eat at aid stations. My goals were to finish in under twenty-four hours and beat four or five horses participating in a concurrent one-hundred-mile horse-endurance race. At mile ninety-three, I sat down (for the first and only time during the race) to drink a cup of soup and got up quickly. John remarked, much to my surprise, "That's good! You were only sitting for two and a half minutes. Now, let's get going." The last seven miles in the deeply forested East Coast mountains were especially dark and difficult. Upon finishing and meeting both my goals, I felt a sense of excitement and amazement at my accomplishment. I had run one hundred miles in twenty-three hours, nineteen minutes, and thirty-six seconds and placed tenth woman in the race. I realized I probably wouldn't have met either goal without the incredible assistance and support from John and others along the way. I considered them all my ultrarunning family. I remain eternally grateful for John teaching me to appreciate companionship.

Diana López, who won a bronze medal in taekwondo at the 2008 Olympics, grew up in an incredibly supportive household. Her parents, Julio and Ondina López, emigrated from Nicaragua to the United States in 1972, and they taught Diana and her three older brothers taekwondo from an early age. Eventually, their oldest brother, Jean, became their coach, with Steven, Mark, and Diana as the competitors. At the 2008 Beijing Olympics, Diana, Steven, and Mark made history as the first trio of siblings to compete in the Olympics since 1904—and as the first trio ever to include a woman. Diana honored her mother during Proctor & Gamble's "Thank You, Mom" at the 2012 Olympics, saying, "She's always said to give it your best. And always finish what you start." She and her brothers remain training partners. The siblings have the same goals and dreams, aiming to be the best that they can be. They carry this motto into their taekwondo academy in Texas. Girls and women, you may not be headed to the Olympics, but you can still train with dedication, focus, and determination like an Olympian, especially with a supportive and loving family around you.[10]

TEN FAMILY STRATEGIES FOR SUPPORTING A YOUNG FEMALE ATHLETE

1. Provide active support in her sport.
2. Encourage siblings to support one another, whether in sports or other activities.
3. Encourage her to make friends with girls on her teams and to have athletic friends.
4. Allow her to establish her own goals and objectives, possibly with your guidance (if requested).
5. Share your own past athletic experiences with her.
6. Check in with her regularly to make sure she's still having fun playing sports.
7. Attend her games, races, meets, or events whenever possible.
8. Be supportive and nonconfrontational in critiquing her athletic performance.

9. If she wants you to, help debrief her after her games, meets, or events.

10. Encourage her to be fully committed, work hard, and do her best.

4

ATHLETIC MOMS' CHALLENGES

Motherhood is a challenging time in an athletic female's life. In the past decades, many professional athletes who wanted to have children often felt compelled to retire. Today, we know better. Research and experience show that sports and exercise are helpful and healthy for both mom and baby. Researchers have discovered that postpartum females experience brain growth that may help them in their mothering. In today's world, many researchers and female athletes believe that childbirth and parenting help women improve as competitive athletes.

Dr. James Pivarnik of Michigan State University has found that women's blood volume increases by 60 percent during pregnancy, possibly improving the body's ability to pass oxygen to the muscles by as much as 30 percent. In the 1980s, East German coaches were rumored to have their female Olympic athletes get pregnant and then abort in order to derive the benefits of the hormones secreted in pregnancy. Theoretically, pregnancy builds up hormonal "effects to create natural blood doping." Some of the areas of improvement include hormonal and physical shifts, as well as a full range of mental changes. To break down these categories even further, researchers observe changes in muscle strength, tolerance of sleep deprivation, endurance, motivation, and overall mental toughness. [1]

Olympic and professional athletic moms, before, during, and after sport, face interesting challenges. The complexity of their juggling act is enormous. They have to train and travel. They have to compete and fight for sponsorships. We're watching the media begin to talk about the issues these athletic moms confront. They have to be mom, partner, and pro athlete. A large study examining working moms' satisfaction concluded that "moms who view their job as a career . . . are more satisfied and feel more positive at work and at home." The Working Mother Research Institute surveyed more than forty-six hundred stay-at-home and working moms, childless women, working fathers, and childless men for this study. Quite likely, career athletic moms experience higher stress levels but greater satisfaction due to their sports passion.[2].

In a 2012 *Washington Post* article, Petula Dvorak jokingly points out that "maybe childbirth and child rearing are the best training for Olympic competition."[3] Research by Dr. Dave Ellemberg has revealed that exercise helps not only mom but baby as well.[4] Apparently, the increase in oxygen, blood volume, and brain activity in mom directly affects baby. This results in brain growth and strengthening for both. In addition, Ellemberg's research points further to an effect on the memory and attention of babies inside the womb.[5]

We are entering an era when competitive female athletes give birth, enjoy their infants, and return wholeheartedly to competition at all levels in most sports. In 1994, pioneers such as Alex Allred broke all the rules and showed what pregnant athletes can actually accomplish. She was a bobsledder who won the National Bobsledding Championship and made the Olympic team at four and a half months pregnant. In 1997, at the top of her game, Sheryl Swoopes, a high-profile basketball player, made headlines. In 1996, she and the US women's basketball team had just garnered gold at the Atlanta Olympics. She followed this by signing a contract with the Houston Comets as part of the inaugural season of the Women's National Basketball Association in conjunction with a lucrative sponsorship with Nike to release a version of basketball shoes called Air Swoopes. She discovered shortly after signing her contract and the shoe deal that she was pregnant. Instead of cancelling her contract, the team kept her on, marketed her as an "everyday mom," and brought her back to work out with the team just six weeks after she gave birth. The team focused on her pregnancy as the family aspect of women's pro basketball. She was able to play the last third of that inaugural season.

PHYSICAL CHALLENGES

According to the old way of thinking, exercise was not recommended for athletic women during their pregnancies. Doctors now tell all pregnant women that moderate exercise three times per week leads to a healthier and more enjoyable pregnancy. Numerous studies support this recommendation. Exercising through your pregnancy can help both you and your baby. Today, professional athletes can train throughout most of their pregnancy at reduced levels of intensity, and they will often return to training in a relatively short time after giving birth. Although there are physical challenges to overcome, female athletes who face uncomplicated pregnancies or who are not at high risk can train well into their pregnancies and recover relatively quickly, participating in training and eventually competing.

Two examples of such women are British marathon runner Paula Radcliffe and former Belgian tennis champ Kim Clijsters. In 2008, ten months after giving birth to her second child, Isla, Paula Radcliffe won the New York City Marathon for a second time. Her primary advice is that "you need a supportive partner—and a baby that sleeps well."[6] Previously ranked (number two) tennis player Kim Clijsters took 2007 to 2009 off to have a baby. When she won the 2009 US Open, she brought baby Jada Elle (eighteen months old) down from the stands to help her celebrate. Kim was the first mother to win a major tennis championship since Evonne Goolagong twenty-nine years previously. Kim and Jada both received Kim's trophy with wide smiles and sparkling eyes.

More recently, two American marathon runners come to mind, Kara Goucher and Deena Kastor. In 2011, at the Boston Marathon, Kara Goucher set a personal best time in the marathon just seven months after giving birth. The following year, Deena Kastor, a 2004 bronze Olympic marathon medalist, finished sixth at the 2012 marathon trials. Her sixth-place finish was remarkable, given that she had an extremely difficult pregnancy and had not run a marathon in over two years. These are just a couple of examples of pro women who've regained their stride and come back even stronger after becoming moms.

"Motherhood changes you because it literally changes a woman's brain—structurally, functionally, and, in many ways, irreversibly."[7] Pregnant women's hormones change in significant ways. The progesterone, estrogen, and oxytocin levels rapidly rise. These hormone changes can often cause disruptions in sleep. As discussed previously, pregnancy increases blood flow, oxygen-carrying capacity, and levels of growth hormone. Specifically through the increase in oxytocin levels, moms develop a greater sensitivity, resulting in a more protective and aggressive stance toward others with regard to their babies. But two of the hormones that increase with pregnancy, testosterone and relaxin, may actually assist females in their athletic capabilities. Testosterone promotes physical strength, and relaxin prepares the body for birth and allows for greater flexibility and joint maneuverability.

We also see a shrinking memory as the belly expands, leading to "mommy brain," a state when mom operates in a sleep-deprived, scattered, and forgetful fog. The difficulties encountered directly relate to hormonal changes that affect the cognitive processes. Specific physical problems that occur include struggles with memory, focus, attention, and visual-spatial tasks. This state of mommy brain often impacts a female athlete throughout her pregnancy. During this time, her mental acuity may feel off, but it does not permanently change her brain. Dr. Jane Martin stresses, "When you are not getting enough sleep and are multitasking, nobody's memory is good. . . . You are not cognitively sharp when you haven't slept well."[8] Despite Dr. Louann Brizendine's estimate that in the first year after birth women lose up to seven hundred hours of sleep, athletic women used to specific training and tasks to take care of themselves and excel in their respective sports suggest that, with easier babies, sleep deprivation doesn't have to interfere nearly as much as predicted. In the last six to twelve weeks of pregnancy, a woman's brain may actually shrink, but it usually begins to recover quickly in the months following pregnancy. Due to the focus that being a mom and athlete requires, we are watching an amazing increase in memory, focus, and attention among athletic moms in shorter periods following childbirth.

According to neuroscientist Dr. Pilyoung Kim, her group of researchers discovered hormonal changes after birth, such as increases in estrogen, oxytocin, and prolactin. These often help mothers' brains to shift and adapt in their responses to their new babies. Sometimes the grey matter—part of the central nervous system, which involves itself in muscle control and sensory perception—even increases in female athletes. We now see high-level athletes training late into their pregnancies and often returning to training within five to ten weeks after giving birth. Particularly in running, we watch women showing great strides in strength and speed.

Their level of fitness is so high that the increase in grey matter often assists in their return to sport more quickly with even better performance than prior to pregnancy. Eventually, they may even develop a higher level of focus and energy for their children and sport. Average athlete moms can also look to return to sport much sooner than previously believed. But the question remains: Does the brain change the behavior, or vice versa, or both? I suspect some of both.[9]

IMPORTANT ASPECTS OF ATHLETIC MOMS' MINDS

Pregnancy brings swift change in emotions. Some female athletes handle this better than others. Some athletes will approach the change in overdrive; others take the time to approach it more slowly. Emotionally and practically, female athletes (like most moms) depend more on others during this period, especially after their babies are born. Yes, their lives will be forever changed, and there is no perfect way to make these changes in lifestyle. In addition to training, they must incorporate time for their babies. One of the primary advantages athletic moms enjoy is their mental fortitude and ability to tolerate high levels of physical discomfort and pain. Olympic, pro, and elite amateur female athletes are used to pushing their bodies to extraordinary physical limits in which their minds play a significant role.

When looking at how the mind works during sport and pregnancy, we see a change in thought processes as motherhood approaches for athletes, especially more hard-core, extreme athletes. For now retired Mountain Bike Hall of Fame professional downhill mountain bike racer Marla Streb (forty-eight), pregnancy and motherhood took her on a distinctly different course of thinking and created a whole new meaning in her life. Her motto had always been "Enjoy it now before you get eaten by worms and bugs." Marla had even dropped out of a PhD program doing AIDS research at Scripps Institute in San Diego to become a professional mountain bike racer. Prior to having children, her fearlessness and risk taking were famous. She was brilliant and a force to be reckoned with—and had numerous broken bones to prove it. In just a two-year span, she broke her collarbone six different times (five seriously), and she sometimes raced with injuries. Her high tolerance for pain was widely known.

One of her competitors, Giove Donovan, simply stated, "Marla's got major *huevos*." Growing up with four brothers, Marla was a rough-and-tumble kind of girl who developed into the same type of adult. She thrived on the thrill of taking extreme risks, including racing down an icy bobsled track in Italy or through a mineshaft in East Germany, where she couldn't see a thing outside the light provided by her headlamp. For Marla, these races provided challenges and got her adrenalin going—at least until she had children.

At forty-two, Marla rode her mountain bike until she was nine months pregnant with her first daughter, Nico, right up until her water broke. Just five weeks after giving birth, she went on to finish third overall at the NORBA National Series event in Vermont. She reflected, "I never used to worry about my personal safety, but after having children I do. . . . As a female athlete, psychologically having to overcompensate creates a tug of war in my mind every second riding. I wanted to win but then you're mom trying to take care of this baby." Her mixed feelings about competing and her role as a mother clearly confused her. Pulled in two different directions, she felt like she was training halfway but still expressed that she spent too much time away from Nico. Her thinking was, "You win or lose in your helmet." Marla clearly believed in the strength of her mental abilities in competition and life in general. She encompassed the athletic woman with both brains and bronze.

Shortly following the birth of her second baby girl, Kiki, Marla finished second and third, respectively, in the Super D and Downhill Nationals in Vermont. At that point, she realized she was done with racing, partially due to the importance she put on being a good mother for her two girls. Marla's commitment to being a mom was quite evident when she pulled up on one of her fun and funky bike designs with baby daughter Nico at our first interview near the Sausalito waterfront. Not much of a car person, she designed and built these funky bikes to accommodate one and then two daughters as she got around town. Marla retired from mountain bike racing and moved to Costa Rica with her husband, Mark, and two girls to design mountain bike parks. Mark has always supported Marla's quirky nature. Now, they live in the Baltimore area, closer to family and Marla's mother, who has Parkinson's disease.

When games, events, races, or matches are close, the emotional mindset of the individual or team can make the difference between winning and losing. Once female athletes' children are born, the organization of their lives will certainly have to tighten up. Nancy Lopez, a pioneering and famous American professional golfer, had three daughters during her professional career and advises other female athletes to prepare to be as organized as possible. A frequent theme heard from these elite athletes involves the considerable reduction of training time. They need to arrange for child care or take their children with them to train. The focus on the quality of workouts takes on paramount importance. They no longer have the luxury of large amounts of time to train, especially those still breast-feeding at two-hour intervals or taking the time to pump breast milk.

Emma Garrard, a thirty-two-year-old top XTERRA pro triathlete, was initially stunned to find out she was pregnant, but she ended up welcoming her pregnancy and child. For her blog, Danelle Kabush, a Canadian Luna XTERRA pro triathlete, interviewed Emma Garrard about her un-planned pregnancy, adjustments, and return to racing. Emma conveyed to Danelle just how emotionally difficult it was dealing with the pregnancy. Both the surprise and concern about her career provided extra stress, but her plan was to have kids during her pro racing career anyway. Her pregnancy just happened sooner than she expected, but she was happy that it came during her thirties. She told Danelle, "I knew my life would not be the same again but knew racing could be an option as there are so many successful athlete-moms out there. . . . It was really stressful making the call to sponsors but they were all very understanding."[10]

Emma continued racing until ten weeks before giving birth, although a good part of that time she was unaware of the pregnancy. She researched exercise and pregnancy, continuing to train with less intensity. In fact, she went into labor right after a swimming pool workout in December 2012. Following her son Torin's birth, her life became all about balance. Between raising Torin, spending time with Ian (her boyfriend), doing more targeted training, competing in fewer races, and performing her other jobs, she works tirelessly to keep things in balance and has support from family and friends. In another interview with GOTRIbal, Emma de-scribed the resources she has accessed to be a stronger and healthier athletic woman: "A supportive family. A community of athletes, particularly other female athletes and especially those I compete against. A good partnership with my sponsors where they believe in what I am doing and I can be a good ambassador for their products."[11] Emma manages to do it all so well that she achieved a podium finish by placing fifth at the October 2013 World XTERRA Championships. She asked for and received loads of assistance from her boyfriend and her family. Her advice for new moms: "Be patient and enjoy being a new mom as the races will always be there."[12]

Female athletes who achieve in their respective sports especially need supportive and engaging partners. Former professional golfer Nancy Lopez recommends, "You have to be with someone who really understands and helps you with the kids." Her words echo the sentiments expressed by marathoner Paula Radcliffe and many other female athletes (both pro and amateur). Part of the task for athletic females is to evolve into their new identity as an athletic mom. Athletic moms need to focus on their children, their training and competition, and making time for their partners. The easier partners make it for them, the more likely the athletic mom's sports success. This involves increased responsibility, focus, and creative organization. Often, stress plays a major role throughout the pregnancy and beyond, but there are numerous options to manage it effectively. Only when partners are threatened by an athletic mom's primary focus on her new child, training, and athletic success do problems occur. This is particularly true among heterosexual husbands and wives.

As in competition, female athletic moms need to acknowledge the role emotions play in their relationships with their babies and children. With many hormonal shifts occurring during and after childbirth, athletic moms need to keep their communication lines open. Since women are primarily "tenders and befrienders," we often feel protective of our children and long for support from other athletic mothers. From the numerous studies on the female brain, we understand that there are psychological and physiological reasons for our need to talk to one another. This is a time when we desire and require more verbal contact than ever before. We need that "relationship dialogue." It's so natural for women to look for collaboration and bonding.

Recently, I interviewed a recreational running mom athlete, Maili Costa. She started running three years ago. Having moved to Marin from San Francisco's East Bay, she has discovered running as a social outlet. She enjoys the talking aspect of running in a group and the "relationship dialogue" with other moms. When the moms compare notes about the struggles athletic moms encounter, Maili focuses on one issue in particular: guilt about whether she's being a good mom and wife. The guilt may surface in the following instances: coming home from running and feeling tired, taking a nap, and worrying about whether she shows up enough for her kids. As thorough organizers, Maili and her husband, Devon (a collegiate and current competitive athlete), work together to make it all work in terms of sports training for both of them. Despite this, Maili and other moms grapple with guilt about the time athletics takes away from their children. Just talking about those feelings can help.

In all the interviews with and research on athletic moms, the sense of connection and bonding with their babies and children is abundantly clear. How women think and feel about themselves and various situations is crucial in managing stress around pregnancy, meeting the many demands of motherhood, and returning to sport. They also find ways to incorporate their children into training, such as through baby joggers or baby bike attachments.

BUILDING BACK YOUR MENTAL SKILLS

While mothering and training, focusing on positive rather than negative thoughts will help athlete moms' performance both as moms and athletes. Look at what you do accomplish rather than what you don't. Acknowledge your past successes in competition and life. Remind yourself that you can strive to return to your previous form. Look at the example of Dara Torres. In 2007, just fifteen months after giving birth to daughter Tessa Grace, Torres medaled in her fifth and final Olympics at age forty-one. Nowadays, more moms are bringing their children to their competitions as she did. Female athletes, in ever increasing numbers, are successfully interrupting training and returning to compete in the same or even better shape than before getting pregnant.

Primary mental skills are confidence, motivation, focus, and concentration, which are all challenges as new moms return to training and eventually competition. To build your confidence, remember the strength it took to adapt to, train during, and enjoy your pregnancy, then to re-emerge and rebuild your life in a whole new way. If you're feeling postpartum blues, just remember that it takes courage to ask for help, so don't be afraid to do so. A common way to motivate yourself is to arrange with your partner to rise early and get out to train or to establish a training partner as you set up a goal to shoot for. If on a team, gradually work yourself into working out with teammates again. As you focus on your new baby, also spend some time on yourself so that you can return to the sport you feel passionate about. Concentrate and organize your schedule to provide positive baby and mom time. Whether concentrating on your little one or sports, commit to being present 100 percent.

COMMITTED STRONG MOM ATHLETES

Alison Dunlap was a two-time Olympic road (1996) and mountain bike (seventh in 2000) racer and is a 100 percent committed pro. In 1999, she rode cross-country mountain bike in the Pan American Games, winning the gold medal. Her athletic accomplishments are too numerous to list here. Held in awe by many, she is a down-to-earth person and was a fierce competitor. Her mind has always been sharp as a tack and strong. She started wanting to have kids during her mid-thirties when her sister had a child, but her husband, Greg Frozley (a former mountain bike racer), wasn't ready as he was concerned about her demanding lifestyle as a pro athlete. Commitment became an issue for Olympian Alison and Greg. He recognized her incredible level of intensity when she approached anything and worried about how she would handle both. Due to an injury resulting in a fourth-degree shoulder separation, she retired for the first time in 2005.

Although she began coaching and started an adventure camp with her husband, Alison returned for a brief stint with Team Luna Chix, racing cyclo-cross in 2009 and 2010. In 2010, she proudly stood up at the Luna Chix Summit and announced to hundreds of women that she was "knocked up." Her excitement was infectious. She had promised her husband that she was done racing and frequently traveling. She was ready to be a mom and to work part-time. Initially, Alison was most surprised by the all-consuming job of taking care of "little Emmett." She has accomplished her goal to create a balance in her life, but her primary focus remains "this little child we've created." Today, she continues to enjoy her three-year-old son, coaches, and works part-time running their adventure camps.

Our natural strengths lie in collaboration, bonding, talking, intuition, empathy, self-control, and concern, according to numerous brain studies.[13] These qualities are important for new moms to draw upon. Cooperation and a desire to bond emotionally in your relationships are qualities that all female athletes, particularly moms, have embedded in their hormonal pool. You will embrace your natural self when you practice these qualities. Female athletes still seem to struggle with how to cooperate and compete. As female athletes, we need to practice both skills. As Emma Garrard has suggested, lean on fellow athletes rather than just family and friends.

Since females are highly verbal creatures, female athletes need to constantly talk things out, especially their emotional issues. Talking helps moms to think problems through and work them out within themselves. Work on cooperating with teammates, other athletic moms, and anyone else who helps you out. Rely on these strengths. Work on trusting your intuitive capabilities. Incorporate empathy and concern into your daily thoughts. Your strong ability to control and organize your lives is a quality that comes in handy before, during, and after pregnancy. One of the common themes that you hear from competitive athletic moms is the need for tighter organization in their lives in order to be good moms, get adequate training, and remain competitive. This skill will help both your baby and yourself. Don't be afraid to show your compassion to yourself and others.

EVOLUTION OF ATHLETIC MOMS AND THEIR CHILDREN

Although Sheryl Swoopes (basketball) had been a groundbreaker in the late 1990s, athletic women in the early 2000s were cautious about mixing pregnancy and sport. The shift toward more relaxed and determined attitudes about having children during their sporting careers has only taken hold among female athletes in recent years.

1980s

Although there were Olympic and pro athletic moms in the 1980s, there is limited information about their athletic life combined with pregnancy and motherhood. During a conversation with a sixty-three-year-old female runner, Charlene Bayles, at the aid station of a running race where we volunteered, she shared with me details about raising her kids in the 1980s while she was a regular runner and worked a demanding full-time job as a clinical research coordinator at the University of California, San Francisco (UCSF). Charlene began running in 1980 during the running craze at that time. Two years after she began running, she became pregnant with her first child. Despite the conventional wisdom at the time that exercise during pregnancy was both unhealthy and dangerous, Charlene ignored these warnings and ran through her second trimester, then switched to swimming when running became difficult. She continued to swim until about a week before she had her son. Then she put him in some sort of a baby jogger and continued her running. During the week, she ran at lunchtime with a group of strong women, including Joan Ulliot and Joan Ottaway (well-known Bay Area runners), who worked at UCSF.

1990s

In the late 1990s, one groundbreaking athlete, Sheryl Swoopes, began the trend in changing attitudes about female athletes, pregnancy, and new mothers' returning to sport. As mentioned in the introduction, the seed for this book was planted in 1994, but my interviews didn't start until 1998. I had been involved in ultrarunning since 1990, so I put out a flyer advertising "female ultrarunners wanted to interview." One woman, Kathy Winkler, agreed to let me interview her although she was primarily a triathlete. In 2013, I was lucky enough to interview her again.

When I first met Kathy, she was a mom, kindergarten teacher, and in her first marriage. A native of Marin County, California, Kathy grew up with many friends who were athletes, especially swimmers and runners. She had participated in one Ironman, at which she had passed out on the run from heatstroke. Two months before Mattie, her oldest daughter, was born in 1992, she went to Tahoe to participate as a backup swimmer in the Trans Tahoe Relay, but no team would take her due to her pregnancy. Just three years later, six weeks after having JoJo, Kathy won the inaugural and short Tiburon Triathlon in 1995 with a half-mile swim, twelve-mile bike ride, and two-mile run. As she raised her daughters and worked full-time as a teacher, she often included the girls in her workouts. Mattie and JoJo rode in baby joggers, then rode bikes alongside while mom ran, and paddled in a canoe while Kathy swam.

Kathy encouraged her daughters to participate in sports of their choice, mainly swimming. Both girls were swimmers, specializing in breaststroke. As Kathy became highly competitive in triathlons with the assistance of local Marin County, California, coach Duane Franks, the girls excelled in sports as well. Kathy's improving success as a triathlete evidently interfered with her first marriage. In 2002, Kathy and her husband split up. The girls lived mainly with her, competing on school and club swimming teams. In 2007, Kathy and her daughters all came together to participate in the Escape from Alcatraz Triathlon, sweeping their respective age groups. A friendly and positive person, Kathy has thrived as an athlete, as have her girls. She made it a point to go to their swimming meets and had them attend her races. When asked how she managed the mom, teacher, and elite amateur athlete roles simultaneously, she depicted her tight organization. Specifically, she always supported her daughters' athleticism, carried sport clothing and equipment in her car, and only did relatively local races (except Ironman Hawaii); her parents helped pick up the slack. Both girls participate in college swimming. JoJo is at the University of California, Los Angeles, and swam in the 2012 Olympic trials. Mattie attends Whittier College, where she swims and plays water polo. Kathy's advice for athletic mothers is to pursue their passion and be a role model for their kids. "I think the most important part of this is the journey and all the incredible people you meet along the way."

TEN MENTAL STRATEGIES FOR ATHLETIC MOMS

1. Join social-networking sites such the Facebook page "Athlete Moms." Connect with mom athletes online at https://www.facebook.com/groups/athletemoms.
2. Actively communicate with your partner and ask for help.
3. Reach out for assistance from friends and families when you need it.
4. Give yourself time to decompress.
5. Connect with other mom athletes locally through sports teams, gyms, and other athletic venues.
6. Train or work out as you feel equipped to do and as advised by a doctor during and after pregnancy. Allow for breaks in training when necessary.
7. Use calming activities to feel centered (e.g., meditation, positive thoughts, yoga).
8. Allow your new identity as mom and athlete to evolve gradually.

9. Encourage your children to participate in sports as they grow older.
10. Think of yourself as an athlete mom.

5

ROMANTIC RELATIONSHIPS

At the recent 2014 Winter Games in Sochi, women made up 105 out of 223 Olympians on the US team. There are now more female athletes competing in sports and more athletic couples with a significant female athlete than ever. Athletic couples include those in which one or both partners are athletes. It has taken a long time for men to accept women as serious competitors. Things have changed though. These days, younger men seem to enjoy supporting their athletic female partners. Still, some athletic women find themselves learning independence and self-sufficiency at a young age, and they may not realize their need for support from others, especially from their romantic partners. When you speak with older female athletes, including Olympians and pros, you will frequently hear that they never even think about the differences between themselves and their male or female counterparts when it comes to how they approach competition and what kind of support system they need. I'm a prime example of this mentality. As a pre–Title IX competitive athlete with extremely critical coaches, I took years to understand my need for support from others, especially my romantic partners, in my sporting activities and in my life. Since my mid-thirties, however, all of my romantic relationships have involved athletic men who have supported my strength and applauded my mental fortitude. My husband, JP, to whom I have been married for thirteen years, has been the most supportive by far. When we met he told me he first noticed me at the end of a Davis Double Century bike ride when I came in ahead of his group. In other words, he noticed me in large part because of my athleticism, which felt like the highest compliment I could have received from him.

We've already discussed the psychological and biological differences between men and women, and it's easy to understand how those differences might come into play in a romantic relationship between a man and a woman. But what about when it's two women in a relationship? As members of the same sex, they have more similarly wired brains; there is a stronger natural basis for them to support and care for one another. After all, our role as females has consisted of naturally falling into caretaking for our men/women in sport. This makes it more likely that athletic women in same-sex relationships will get the type of support they need from their partners, though, of course, every relationship is different.

Lesbians often provide a lot of support for each other. The number one pick in 2013's professional women's basketball draft, Brittney Griner, talked publicly and openly about being gay. She was open about this even during her college years playing at Baylor, although no public announcement was ever made. Brittney's girlfriend is the one topic that she is not open about. You hear only snippets about her relationship, such as rumors that her parents now e-mail her girlfriend. In contrast, Megan Rapinoe, an Olympic and World Cup USA soccer player, is open about her relationship with Sarah Walsh, a pro Aussie soccer player, which has been going on for more than four years. Distance has not created a problem for the pair. Rapinoe says, "Most people who are in a relationship on our team, it's basically long distance, because we're gone so much. . . . You have to have the right personality to go the distance we go and go the time we go. It's not for everyone."[1] According to Walsh, "We make fun of each other a lot and one of the things I love about her is that she can make fun of herself. People are drawn to her."[2]

HOW THE SEXES VALUE RELATIONSHIPS DIFFERENTLY

As Dr. Deborah Tannen discovered years ago, women are drawn to emotional intimacy and men to independence. Men think of relationships from a cognitive and analytical perspective, primarily engaging in activity-based relationships, and this is especially true in athletics. "Communication is a continual balancing act," Tannen writes, involving "juggling the conflicting needs for intimacy and independence." In terms of sports, this means that women approach competition with an emotional component that directly impacts their response to the outcome of a given event. Whether they are satisfied with that outcome or not, female athletes are likely to carry at least some of the emotions sparked during competition with them when they walk off the field, court, or track.

SUPPORTIVE SECOND PARTNERS

Since relationships are first and foremost on female athletes' priority lists, the key to their having a successful relationship is a partner who expresses support for their participation in their sport and for their need for cooperation, collaboration, and bonding. This is especially important for male partners to understand because men generally operate in a more hierarchical and cognitive style. Many female athletes who got their start during the early days of Title IX (and who have since been divorced and remarried) cite a lack of support in their first marriage, particularly regarding their sport, as the reason for its failure. In order for a couple to succeed, then, they have to work together to understand and accept each other's style. For most women this probably means talking a lot, since that is the main way that they communicate. But this won't necessarily come naturally to most men, particularly when it comes to discussing the relationship. The more positive spoken communication between any couple, however, the better, especially if one of the partners involved is a female athlete.

Dr. Christine Thorburn, 2004 and 2008 Olympic road cyclist, describes herself as a competitive, stubborn, and focused athlete. She says her first husband was quite controlling and didn't want her to race bikes. When she decided to ride in a bike tour from San Francisco to Portland, Oregon, during her sophomore year at Stanford, he tried to talk her out of it, saying she "shouldn't mix medicine and cycling." Christine eventually realized that her marriage was hindering her involvement in competitive athletics and that her husband was not supporting who she was—so she divorced him. Christine met her second husband, Ted Huang, an outgoing and intense engineer who competed in the 1996 Olympics as a windsurfer, through cycling. Christine says that Ted admires her for her athletic prowess, and he always wants to see her succeed. He even significantly helped coach her for the 2008 Olympics. She talked about Ted as her number one supporter and confidant, describing him as supportive, generous, and competitive. He is proud to be the spouse of a female Olympian and doctor, and she trusts him to support her entirely in all endeavors in life, sports related or not. You can often see them riding on the road together in Portola Valley south of San Francisco.

Elite amateur triathlete Jeri Howland and her husband, Jerry Edelbrock, offer another example of a mutually supportive athletic couple. Jeri specializes in triathlons and short ultras (50K and Quad Dipsea), and since 1999 Jerry has received fourteen Dipsea black shirts, earned for making it through the Dipsea Race (the second-oldest foot race in the country, behind only the Boston Marathon) in the top thirty-five. Though training and competing form a big part of their lifestyle, Jeri and Jerry have made a pact rarely to compete in the same event at the same time, though they do attend each other's events as a way of showing support. It's an unusual approach, but it works for them. "Jerry is so proud of me, and has a high tolerance for the large amount of time my training takes as a triathlete," Jeri says. "He lets me shine." Like Christine, Jeri was married once before, to a husband who didn't meet her needs as a female athlete. In Jerry, however, she has found a best friend and competitive equal.

Christine and Jeri both come from a generation in which female athletes were not respected or encouraged, even by their own husbands. Today, however, both women are supported by their second husbands, each of whom is a strong athlete in his own right. Despite their female/ male differences, with love, support, and open communication, these couples have found a way to make things work. It takes persistence and patience, but Christine and Jeri are living proof that it's possible for female athletes to build healthy relationships that will provide them with the support they relish and thrive on.

HOW OUR BRAINS ARE DIFFERENT

As discussed in chapter 1, female brains work differently from male brains. Women are more apt to use both sides of the brain, for example, in contrast to men's tendency to use one. Meanwhile, men's brains are 9 percent larger than women's brains, though females' brains are just as packed with neurons. This is not to say that one gender is better or smarter than the other. Actually, despite their differences, both sexes perform equally well on intelligence tests. However, male and female brains are not built the same way, and as a result men and women use different parts of their brain when tackling certain tasks.

Numerous researchers have discovered that the level of general brain activity in women is much greater than in men, particularly in the areas of language, socializing, bonding, organizing, planning, empathizing, and experiencing relationships from an emotional perspective. In contrast, men value relationships in a more cognitive and analytical style, excelling in visual-spatial tasks and analytic and cognitive information processing; they also have 2.5 times larger sex drives, respond to threats with the fight-or-flight response, and are at greater risk for addiction problems. This is the biological imperative that directs us all to act.

In the past several years, researchers have determined that the prefrontal cortex, which inhibits impulsive behavior and is the area where we deal with anger, fear, and aggression, develops sooner and is larger in women than it is in men. This area is considered the "CEO of the brain" because it is responsible for such functions as decision making, problem solving, and organization. The other areas of the cortex most active in women are the frontal cortex, anterior cingulate, and insular, which are responsible for intuitive feelings and greater self-consciousness. As Dr. Louann Brizendine has commented, "The relationship between a women's gut feeling and her intuitive hunches is grounded in biology." So both sexes have aggression, but because their brains are designed differently, they have different methods of displaying it: women use talking to get their way, whereas men use analytical skills and physical domination. It makes sense, then, that sports provide both women and men with the perfect place to express any aggressive tendencies in a positive manner.[3]

Researchers have discovered five other primary brain areas that function at stronger and more active levels in women than men, including the hippocampus, the far left of the amygdala, the mirror-neuron system, the limbic cortex, and the white matter. The hippocampus is where short-term memories are transformed into long-term memories. The far left of the amygdala, at the base of the hippocampus, plays a large role in emotional, social, and motivational responses. The mirror-neuron system allows women to be more sensitive to the observation and feeling of experiences in events and to react in an emotional way. This actually creates a way for women to "feel" the pain of others and express empathy. The limbic cortex regulates emotions and is much larger in women than men. This means that women can express emotion better than men, but it also puts them at risk for depression and anxiety problems.

The final area of the brain that functions at a more active level in women than in men is the white matter, which connects one part of the brain to another. This allows women to more readily access both sides of the brain and develop organizational skills. In relationships, this translates into females having greater short-term memories, empathy, multitasking skills, and access to emotional, social, and motivational responses than their male counterparts. If both partners are involved in competitive sports, the woman's role in the partnership often involves using these capabilities to help both organize their involvement in athletics within the context of their lives.

In contrast, men's strengths lie in the areas of finding cognitive and analytic solutions to relationship struggles. The stronger-functioning areas of the male brain are the temporal-parietal junction, gray matter, parietal cortex, grey matter hypothalamus, ventral tegmental area, and far right of the amygdala. The parietal-temporal junction directs males to view relationships from a cognitive and analytical perspective. (That is why men often want to "fix" problems in relationships.) The gray matter directly influences information processing, helping men to see more technical details (for example, with bike maintenance in sports). The parietal cortex operates spatial perception, allowing men to exhibit a greater sense of spatial context. (For example, men seem more comfortable than women with riding close in cycling pacelines.) The ventral tegmental area functions as a center for motivation and reward. The far right of the amygdala operates outward actions and external stimuli, such as the fight-or-flight response in reaction to danger and threats. This drives males to protective aggression, like when a football player is unnecessarily manhandled and his teammates rise to his defense. In short, male athletes regard relationships primarily from an analytical and unemotional perspective.[4]

When looking at male-female sporting couples, it's easy to recognize the differences between them. Women show more emotion, memory, empathy, socializing, and multitasking; men, in contrast, are detail oriented, spatially alert, protectively aggressive problem solvers. Simply put, females operate from their hearts; males operate from their thoughts. Male-female athletic couples, like all couples, often find themselves working hard to meet in the middle and appreciate what each other has to offer.

ATHLETIC COUPLE DYNAMICS

Athletic couples' dynamics are vast and varied. Any difficulties that couples encounter in their lives are often magnified when one or both partners play and compete in sports. This is especially the case for women, since they need a certain amount of attention, reassurance, and belief in themselves to perform optimally. Men, in contrast, are generally perfectly fine acting independently in sports. Of course, they do appreciate a certain amount of support as well. The difference here is biologically and culturally based. As discussed, females are emotional and males are cognitive in their relationship focus, and since primary relationships usually hold the most meaning for us, women look heavily to them for support. In ever increasing numbers, we see men attending women's sporting events. Even top competitors look to their partners for backing. For women who are active athletes to be successful and feel satisfied in their relationships, especially if their partners are also athletes, a certain amount of give-and-take is required on both sides.

Honor and Bob Fetherston, a couple with whom my husband and I happen to be friends, are partners who totally support each other in their athletic pursuits. Their relationship is a model for give-and-take. Honor's focus is on running; she was a top US Masters runner in the 1990s. She ran in the 1996 Olympic trials at age forty-one and was named 1995 USA Track & Field 40–44 Master of the Year. Bob, meanwhile, has excelled in doing triathlons, racing road bikes, and participating in long-distance road rides. The couple has long trained together on the track and the road, and the balance they've attained in their relationship is impressive. Whenever Bob participates in long-distance cycling events, Honor is close by in her car, crewing for her husband. I can think of one example in particular. Years ago, when the California Death Ride was three passes, Bob, my husband, and another friend of ours, Terry, were riding the course. In the course of three passes, it rained, snowed, sleeted, and hailed. Honor was there for them at every checkpoint, providing dry clothes, hot drinks, and whatever else they needed. The ride and the crewing that day were epic. And Bob has done the same for Honor: when her talented running skills took her to national status in the 1990s, Bob was right there by her side, supporting her along the way.

TYPES OF ATHLETIC COUPLES

All romantic relationships face a number of challenges, but when the partners involved are both athletes and also work full-time, their lives are more complicated in terms of organization, training, and competing. Athletic training adds a whole other dimension to one's lifestyle. For relationship-oriented female athletes, certain emotional elements require tending from their partners. Generally speaking, men who are not athletes struggle more with addressing these needs than men who are. I've had my own experience with this issue: after becoming a runner and racer, I dated a nonathletic man who just wanted to hover over—rather than help—me all the time. (It was a short-lived relationship.)

Athletic men can also have trouble meeting the needs of their athletic female partners, however. Some expect their partners to adhere to their schedules, and never the other way around, and some struggle with their partners outcompeting them. I once had a partner, Simon, who was a much slower runner than I, but he would try to outpace me anyway. At one point we went on vacation to a tropical island, and while there, we went on daily runs together. Every day, Simon would quickly pick up the pace . . . and then begin to fade. I would continue at the pace he had established, and he would fall behind. When this happened, the island men we passed on our route would harass him, telling him to pick up the pace and catch up, but he couldn't, and he always ended up mad at me. He couldn't accept the fact that we simply had different paces. The relationship was doomed to fail.

Partners in a sports-playing couple should ask themselves a number of questions in order to prevent avoidable problems from cropping up in the relationship:

- Do we compete in the same events, meets, or races? If not, how do we offer support for each other's competitions?
- How do we handle competition, especially if we will potentially be competing against one another?

- How can we create routines to more effectively handle organization? When will each of us train? How will we organize training and competing?
- How will we meet each other's needs despite our busy schedules?
- Will we both try to attend each other's events, or will we go separately?
- How will we include or exclude our children? Will we take turns with child care?

Athletic couples operate in a variety of ways, but through observation and interviews, I have identified five positive models: (1) mutually supportive in the same sport, (2) actively supportive, (3) introduced to sport by partner, (4) quietly supportive, and (5) mutually supportive in different sports. It's important to note that all five of these models involve some form of support. Not every female athlete needs the same kind of support, but all female athletes are more likely to perform at their best when they feel emotionally supported.

Mutually Supportive in the Same Sport

In a mutually supportive relationship, the two partners are both athletes, and they support each other to perform their best through actions and words. Just like any other couple, they may have their ups and downs and disagreements, but they always have each other's back. These couples strategize and discuss their individual sporting goals with one another and work together to realize them. Interestingly enough, I've found that this type of model is a rarity among female athletes; the vast majority of the women I have interviewed over the years do not have partners who are their equal when it comes to competitive sports. The National Basketball Association's Kevin Durant and the Women's National Basketball Association's (WNBA) Monica Wright were officially engaged as of July 2013. They are not a new couple, just a quiet and discreet one. Introduced in 2006 at the all-American high school all-star showcase in San Diego, the couple was described as having a close "friend" relationship but not a romantic one. In addition to their love of basketball, their friendship lays a solid foundation for their future together. When Kevin Durant was asked about how he felt about his fiancée's team, the Minnesota Lynx, winning the 2013 WNBA Championship, he tweeted, "I love it!!! She's the better player anyway . . . and I was proud of how she helped her team win a championship. It was kind of tears of joy."

Barbra Higgins, a Panamanian fencer who competed in the 1984 Olympics, had a mutually supportive relationship during her fencing years. Her partner was also a female Olympic fencer, and their relationship centered on the sport. Barbra's girlfriend, in fact, encouraged her to try out for the Olympics. They even moved to San Francisco together to take advantage of the great coaches in the area—especially San Jose, where Barbra trained—and they built a fencing strip at home so they could spar there. Through their mutual love of fencing and their mutual support, their bonds held strong as long as they were in fencing together.

Samantha Gash, an Australian ultrarunner and qualified attorney, set the record in the Race the Planet seven-day race series as the first and youngest woman to complete the 4 Deserts race series in one year. Samantha and her boyfriend, Mathieu, who's also an endurance runner, met crewing for Catherine Todd, an Australian runner, at the Badwater 135 race that begins in Death Valley, California, and ends at Mount Whitney in California. Samantha and Mathieu enjoy common loves, including endurance running, training, and crewing for others, as well as the enjoyment they derive from their work. Sam focuses on the organization in the relationship, and Mathieu focuses on the balance. She explains, "Mathieu and I are very committed to sharing as many of our interstate/overseas race/travel experiences together. And for the times when we can't physically be there together—we will make sure the other person is a part of the experience as much as possible. I am lucky to share a life with someone who is as committed to the same goals and values as I have."

Jamie Rivers, a local, Marin County-known Dipsea runner, and her husband, Roy, offer another prime example of a mutually supportive couple. Prior to their marriage in 2010, Jamie and Roy trained together with the same group to run the Dipsea Race in Mill Valley, California. Jamie says that she and Roy both gave each other constant support during that time. Jamie also loves that Roy appreciates her lively, upbeat attitude: "Roy is not intimidated by my antics," she says. Her competitive nature matches her husband's, and they both seem to revel in their mutual passion for trail running. In 2007, they finished the handicapped Double Dipsea Race together, arriving at the finish line hand in hand—demonstrating that even in the heat of competition, they stick by each other's side.

Actively Supportive

Actively supportive relationships, in which female athletes are supported and encouraged by their partners (athletic or nonathletic, male or female), are the most common type I've encountered in the pool of female athletes I've interviewed. Actively supportive partners are excited by their partners' athletic successes, whether they are pros, Olympians, or amateurs. Some embrace and get involved with all the prep and training that their partners require to achieve peak performances; others simply make time allowances. Still others help keep their athletic partners' equipment, such as bicycles in road, track, or mountain biking, in prime condition.

Professional mountain bike racer and 2012 London Olympic bronze medalist (in the mountain bike cross-country race) Georgia Gould grew up in an outdoorsy and active family with four brothers. Georgia used the outdoors as her playground. She met her husband, Dusty, when she was working as a waitress in Sun Valley, Idaho. That was fifteen years ago, when Georgia was just eighteen. Dusty is a pro mechanic, and he shows his support for Georgia in a variety of ways. As a mechanic, he has a strong interest in mountain biking and is an amateur athlete himself. Each day, Dusty inquires about how Georgia's training went, and if Georgia is tired from a long training session, he'll pick up dinner. She says he expresses his love for her, admiration for her hard work ethic, and belief in her as a person multiple times a day. In other words, he has her back. When the chips are down, he is right there by her side, verbally encouraging her. He also gives her bike lots of TLC and is constantly looking for ways to improve its performance. Georgia's biggest cheerleader at races is Dusty. When I asked her what role relationships have played in her athletic career, Georgia stressed that her support network is of paramount importance to her success as an athlete, and Dusty is the key member of that network.

Just twelve days after they were married in 2008, Brew Davis faithfully followed Jennifer Pharr Davis in a successful bid to break the women's record in speed-hiking the Appalachian Trail. A few years later in 2011, Jennifer decided to speed-hike the Appalachian Trail again in an attempt to break the record for both men and women. Unfortunately, Brew tore his ACL before the hike began, preventing hiking alongside Jennifer as he had planned. However, his love for and dedication to his wife became apparent when, in a T-shirt and jeans and with a heavily bearded face, he emerged constantly along the trail, providing snacks and meals, encouragement, and a place for Jennifer to sleep every night. She had people hiking with her for over 40 percent of the time, from Pennsylvania on, but between Maine and Pennsylvania, where she had no one with her, Brew followed a parallel route along the road. Jennifer later said that relying on her husband and crew significantly contributed to her pain endurance and ability to remain focused in the present moment during the hike.

Rail thin and weathered, Jennifer Pharr Davis finished the final climb to the summit of Spring Mountain, Georgia, on July 31, 2011, having set a new overall (female or male) record of forty-six days, eleven hours, and twenty minutes. Brew accompanied her as she emerged from the woods and climbed onto the granite slab at the top. Her gaggle of fans and supporters clapped, cheered, and clicked photo after photo as Jennifer exclaimed, "We did it! Despite the people who told us we couldn't and against all odds, we believed in one another and we accomplished something amazing." Later, reflecting on the experience, Jennifer said, "I think of this as a love story. . . . The biggest theme for me was how much my husband loved me." Brew was there from start to finish, crewing and providing both emotional and physical support throughout the course, and it made all the difference to Jennifer's success.

Introduced to Sport by Partner

Female athletes introduced to their main sport by their partners are generally women who have previously been outstanding athletes in other sports. Prior to cycling, for example, Meredith Miller played collegiate and even semipro soccer. She even met Ben, her eventual husband, while playing soccer. After they started dating, Ben got Meredith into road cycling so they could cycle together. He began road racing a year prior to Meredith, who entered the fray at age twenty-five, but it was Meredith who eventually evolved into a pro road and cyclo-cross racer. I first interviewed her in 2010, a year after she became the 2009 National Road Race Champion. Meredith said that Ben has been by her side, encouraging, supporting, and expressing pride in her accomplishments, throughout her pro career. She also said he's showed enormous patience for all the traveling that her job entails.

Bay Area couple Lorraine Jarvis and Kelly Silberberg further illustrate this model. Kelly, Lorraine's husband, is a former collegiate track cyclist.

They met playing volleyball, but eventually she started cycling with him, and he nudged her into competing at an elite amateur level with his team, which just happened to need another female teammate. Kelly's support has been key to Lorraine's success. He is her coach and closest confidant. Lorraine is intensely driven and hardworking, and she needs her attention to be completely focused when she's preparing and training for events, so each year she and Kelly put together a structured training schedule to help keep her on track. Lorraine won two world championships in the fifty to fifty-four time trial age group in 2008 and 2009. In 2013, Lorraine and another Bay Area favorite, Julia Violich, joined up and won the national 40K time trial in under an hour, earning them the Women's Tandem 70 and Over National Championship. Lorraine says that Kelly's energy has contributed again and again to her continuing achievements; she describes him as intelligent, thoughtful, encouraging, and calm under pressure. Lorraine is one tough competitor, but she needs support just like any other female athlete when competing, and Kelly meets that need.

Quietly Supportive

Quietly supportive partners are usually not athletes themselves, although some athletes fall into this category. For these types of relationships to work, continuous and clear written and verbal communication is key. Whether the women in these couples are pros or amateurs, their level of competition impacts their lifestyle. Especially with pros, the travel required by sporting competitions and the separation it creates are ongoing factors in a romantic relationship. These couples have to work to stay connected.

Former Canadian Olympic road and track racer Gina Grain met her girlfriend, Anita, a photojournalist, at a race. During the course of Gina's career, her girlfriend wished to remain in the background. On longer training trips and track races in different countries, Anita would occasionally travel with her. She was present when Gina won the silver medal at the world championships in Bordeaux, France, in 2006 and competed in the Olympics in 2008. Since Anita was a sports photojournalist, she also traveled a lot following the race circuit, and Gina connected with her. Gina describes her as "very, very supportive" and encouraging during that time; she simply didn't want to be in the spotlight. In July 2010, Gina retired. In 2013, the couple married.

Mutually Supportive in Different Sports

Since the majority of female athletes meet their partners through sports, their partnerships are more often based in the same sport than in different ones. However, couples who compete in different sports do exist, and for partners who fall into this category, cooperation and collaboration is essential to their success.

The most widely recognized and talked about sports couple of 2013 included famous golfer Tiger Woods and Lindsey Vonn, an American World Cup alpine ski racer. They support each other by attending each other's sports competitions: Lindsey supported Tiger by attending tournaments during the summer, and Tiger attended a World Cup race Lindsey competed in. Olympic gold medalist track-and-field athlete Sanya Richards-Ross and NFL cornerback Aaron Ross, who played for the Giants during two Super Bowl wins, are another example of a mixed-sports couple. They started as college sweethearts at the University of Texas, and their relationship is still going strong. Before the 2012 London Olympics, Aaron commented, "I love to see her run," and he got permission from the Jacksonville Jaguars to attend the 2012 London Olympics to watch his sprinter wife compete. He watched her win gold in the four hundred meter. As she ran to him in the stands after the win, Aaron exclaimed, "You finally did it, babe. Enjoy the moment." Aaron is the laid-back member of this couple; he usually lets Sanya, the firebrand, get her way. Sanya's most recent idea was their new reality TV show, *Sanya's Glam & Gold*, in the summer of 2013.

Female athletes' primary relationships are clearly critical to their success in sports. Through open communication, emotional and other forms of support, bonding, collaboration, and romantic partners can play a huge role in helping female athletes achieve their competitive desires and goals. Their partners' verbal and physical presence can be important to female athletes as they train and compete to achieve success. Their success stems from, among others things, setting goals, achieving them, and having the support of a romantic relationship.

TEN MENTAL STRATEGIES FOR SUPPORTING THE FEMALE ATHLETE IN YOUR LIFE

1. All female athletes need intimate emotional support, even if they deny it.
2. Communication for women is best accomplished through talking.
3. Cooperation, collaboration, and bonding are all key for women.
4. Approach your female partner from a positive perspective.
5. Female athletes may be more intuitive, decisive, and self-conscious than their male counterparts.
6. Attention, reassurance, and encouragement help female athletes achieve personal records (PRs).
7. Mutually collaborative and supportive relationships work the best for women.
8. Provide feedback while assuring your female athlete she is the number one person in your life.
9. A strong, positive athletic identity is essential for female athletes.
10. A partner needs to treat the female athlete with respect and admiration for her to perform at her personal athletic best.

6

BODY IMAGE OF FEMALE ATHLETES

What is body image? Body image consists of the internalized thoughts, feelings, and attitudes a girl or woman has about her body and how she thinks that others perceive her. It further pertains to a female's perception of her outward physical appearance, including weight, size, and body shape. Our culture focuses on what women's bodies look like, while sports focus on what women's bodies can do. Because of this, playing sports can improve women's body image; however, females in sports do still struggle with the cultural and social ideal emphasizing thinness over strength and differing athletic body types.

During the 2012 London Olympics, a senior UK athletics official described the diminutive 5'5" Jessica Ennis-Hill, a heptathlete and member of the British Olympic track-and-field team, as "fat," disregarding the fact that her particular sport requires muscular strength and endurance. Ennis-Hill ignored the remark and went on to become a gold medalist in the 2012 Olympic heptathlon. But this is just one of many instances in which people, particularly men, in the sports world have evaluated female athletes' bodies by their looks rather than their performance ability.

Female athletes also face "sports body stereotypes" within particular sports. I've faced this issue myself. Years ago, when I was thin as a rail for my endomorphic and muscular body type, I ran my first marathon in a total state of fitness in San Francisco. After the race was over, people commented that I didn't "look like a marathon runner." The perception was clearly that only tiny, exceedingly thin women were true marathoners. They didn't understand that thinness does not necessarily equal fitness and health. For evidence of this, just look at the Williams sisters. They are big, strong, powerful women. Their bodies don't fit our society's ideal of thinness; nor do they fit what many might view as the "typical" body profile for female pro tennis players. But between them, they've dominated the tennis world since they were young teens, winning ten Wimbledon championships in recent history.

BASICS OF BODY IMAGE

Body image begins to form in early childhood and is influenced by both nature and nurture. It's long been clear that how your parents raise you to regard people's physical appearance, both your own and others', directly impacts how you think and feel about your body. A mother's body image may especially influence her daughter's perception of her own body. Foremost, our relationships with other people influence our body image. Even statements by coaches, such as, "You're getting fat," can sometimes trigger girls to develop eating disorders. More current research, however, points to temperament as being part of the equation as well.[1] Females who are naturally prone to high anxiety, self-consciousness, obsessiveness, and perfectionism are more likely to experience body image issues and concerns than those who are not.

Many women who have become competitive athletes were considered tomboys as children, grew up in families that emphasized sports, or were raised around brothers. These athletic girls used to be considered "unladylike," a perception that significantly affected their body images. Pre–Title IX female athletes were often seen as more fragile, and their mothers often restricted their athletic participation. That type of thinking has rapidly declined in the years since the passage of Title IX in 1972. Interestingly, Title IX was originally designed to provide equal educational opportunities for girls and boys in high school and college, and the inclusion of sports was merely one small component of the plan. In hindsight, however, the legislation seems to have made the most visible and positive impact in the sports world, and part of that impact has been on female athletes' body image. The Women's Sports Foundation talks about the fact that girls and women who play sports have a more positive body image and are happier psychologically than girls and women who do not play sports.

Ana Braga-Levaggi grew up in Brazil, where, she says, females are self-conscious about their bodies, yet not afraid to let others see them, large and small alike. Most of her family members suffer from weight problems, including her mother, who is a considerably overweight woman. She described her entire family as battling body image issues. Ana moved to the Bay Area in the mid-1980s to learn English, and when she got here, she took up aerobics, eventually going on to manage a health club. She later took up running, and in 1993 she ran her first marathon. Ana says she started running to maintain her weight and improve her body image, something she had long struggled with. Over the years, she says, her perception of her body has changed a couple of times. All through her forties, she ran ultramarathons and felt comfortable with her body. But at age forty-seven, as menopause set in, she noticed that her body was changing and that she had to work harder to maintain her weight. Only now, at fifty-three, after years of struggling to accept some of the changes occurring in her body, has she learned how to embrace her body for what it is.

It's been estimated that up to 80 percent of American women are unhappy with some part of their bodies, be it their butts, thighs, hips, breasts, or something else. I've seen it time and again, even in unexpected places. Years ago, for example, one of the more talented runners in my area, a lithe, petite, rail-thin woman, showed up at a race with giant new breasts that appeared totally out of place then and still do. Even this winning competitive runner was dissatisfied with her body.

It's no secret where at least part of this dissatisfaction comes from. When women compare themselves to the ultrathin models found everywhere from TV to magazines, they are bound to feel inadequate and frustrated and to form negative body images. It's a well-known fact that the vast majority of American women (as many as 98 percent) will never be as thin as supermodels. That doesn't prevent the other 98 percent from striving to look like that 2 percent, however: "Apparently, because dissatisfaction is so prevalent in the US, being a woman and being worried about your body and weight is considered part of being female."[2]

One former ultrarunner, Martha Cederstrom, describes herself as always having been athletic and says she was considered a tomboy in her youth. Her parents, sister, and brother weren't especially athletic, but that didn't discourage Martha. She became a pioneering competitive ultrarunner during the late 1980s, when she was in her thirties. After running her first Western States one-hundred-miler in 1989, missing a silver belt buckle by only seconds, her attitude toward her body began to change. She began to believe that she could do anything she wanted. She liked the lean, muscular look running had given her body, and she became much less self-conscious about her looks. Today, Martha says that the strength she gained through ultrarunning helped her and her other ultrarunning girlfriends build self-confidence and improve their body images permanently. She no longer competes in ultrarunning, but she still runs, and she now practices and teaches yoga as well, activities that help her maintain her fitness. It took her years to get to a place where she could embrace her athletic body, but now Martha is comfortable in her own skin—and sports helped her get there.

The Body Positive, a wonderful organization, has established a model for women to follow in order to develop a healthier body image. The model focuses on moving women away from the idea of "perfection" and toward caring for the bodies they have. Its five steps are to (1) reclaim health, (2) practice intuitive self-care, (3) cultivate self-love, (4) declare one's own authentic beauty, and (5) build community. Together, these steps mean exploring the influences that have impacted your relationship with nutrition, exercise, and your body; learning to focus on health rather than weight; learning to trust and pay attention to your body so that you know when you are actually hungry and when you're not and so that you're aware of the type of nutrition your body needs; learning to express yourself in a positive manner and reduce your self-critical thoughts; acknowledging and appreciating your unique beauty, inside and out; recognizing that beauty is an ongoing, ever-transforming process; and connecting with others who see, appreciate, and welcome our differences. This model reminds us of the importance of accepting each other's bodies, and it's one that all female athletes could benefit from using.

WHAT IS A FIT BODY?

How do you view your body? How have all of the people in your life—parents, friends, boyfriends, girlfriends—and the media influenced your confidence in your body's ability to perform? Did your parents praise you for your training and performance in sports? Did they emphasize healthy nutrition as an important part of your sporting activities? Or did your mother constantly try to scare you with threats that you would gain a pound if you took a bite of chocolate cake? Would you father also make comments that made you feel self-conscious? If you're tall, did family members often remind you that you were a big girl, regardless of your dress or pant size? How about your coaches—were they supportive, or did they emphasize the importance of not getting fat and tell you to do whatever it took to look and perform well?

The media's portrayal of what makes a girl or woman good-looking and "fit" is still overly skewed toward thinness, a misrepresentation that makes many female athletes compare themselves unrealistically to these rail-thin role models. Unfortunately, many female athletes' friends, family members, and coaches also hold these misconceptions about what their body size and shape should be, and that damages their self-perception further.

In 1987, when I was running my first marathon, my boyfriend shot a photo of me from the rear. In the picture, running alongside me, there is another woman who has cellulite covering her upper rear legs. When I showed the photo to a girlfriend of mine, she couldn't get past the cellulite on the woman's legs. She just couldn't accept that a woman who looked like that could have run a marathon, let alone in well under four hours. Her inability to view this woman as a serious athlete was clearly a product of the media's insistence on continuing to depict the ideal female athlete's body as thin and flawless and general ignorance of the fact that cellulite is often the result of genetics and has nothing to do with one's ability to engage in sports. And even Olympians have to deal with the ramifications of this false ideal, as evidenced by British female heptathlete Jessica Ennis-Hill's being called "fat."

Today, many big, strong Olympic and professional female athletes—like Serena Williams, Dara Torres (Olympic gold medalist swimmer), Laila Ali (pro boxer), and Elana Meyers (Olympic silver medalist in bobsledding)—are admired for their size, strength, and fitness level. These athletic women are proud of their bodies, as evidenced by their positive attitudes and confidence in themselves, and they are viewed with respect by younger women. As a sports psychologist, I encourage my athletic female clients to use these role models and their inspirational words to help them improve their own body image. In the words of Elana Meyers, "As Olympic athletes, we have a responsibility to be positive role models to today's youth."

Shana Bagley, an amateur, multisport competitor, was raised in San Rafael, California, where her parents still live. Shana competes in nontraditional sports, including strongman, Scottish Highland games, men's rugby, and ocean sailing, all of which require muscular strength and endurance. She is an unusual athlete: in high school, she played on the varsity men's water polo team (a tough, physical sport), and then, after taking years off, she took up competitive sports again in her thirties. When I interviewed Shana in 2009, she had been playing for three years on a men's rugby team that had placed second in the national championship games, and she was about to be a crew member in the Clipper Round the World Yacht Race. Her strength was best displayed, however, when she participated in a strongman competition and pulled a caboose and fire truck.

Shana has a bigger body type, and she's never been what most would consider thin. But her size is part of why she is as strong as she is; if she were model-thin, she could never have pulled a fire truck in a strongman competition. Shana says the competition required not only a lot of physical strength but a lot of mental strength as well. Most importantly, she had to have complete confidence in her body to pull the feat off. She says she's had some issues with body image over the years, but her self-confidence has definitely improved since she started competing in sports again as an adult.

So what is a fit body? A fit body is strong but not necessarily thin or perfectly shaped. The fit female athlete trains hard, eats healthily, and has a positive mental attitude. She is comfortable with her body and fitness, and she believes in herself. But in order for more female athletes to fit this profile, they need to improve their body image, and that means being surrounded by people who support this view of fitness. Positive body image is essential to success in sports and life, and female athletes need help building that image.

DISORDERED EATING AND EATING DISORDERS

Female athletes are at much higher risk for developing disordered eating or eating disorders than the general public. Research consistently shows that one-third of all collegiate female athletes engage in disordered eating or suffer from eating disorders. This is influenced by the sports milieu;

sports that emphasize thinness and weight control have higher incidences of eating disorders.[3] Specifically, sports focused on appearance, judging, agility, weight, and endurance pose a high risk: gymnastics, figure skating, dancing, diving, distance running, cross-country skiing, and synchronized swimming all have a higher percentage of athletes with eating disorders. Female athletes who play sports that require muscle mass and bulk, meanwhile (such as basketball, skiing, heptathlon, and volleyball), are less likely to develop eating disorders.

When you look at the 2012 London Olympic sports such as tennis, soccer, beach volleyball, and basketball, you will observe strong female athletes who don't fit our cultural ideal. It is the more successful female athletes with positive coaching, such as Alison Dunlap (Olympic road, 1996, and mountain biker, 2000) and Misty May-Treanor (Olympic beach volleyball player, 2000, 2004, 2008, and 2012), who express comfort with their body image, confidence, and self-esteem.

Female athletes who struggle constantly with their body image can easily develop disordered eating or eating disorders, especially if they're extremely competitive: "The more competitive people are, even if they're just competitive with themselves, the more likely they are to have the kind of thinking that can lead to disordered eating patterns," says Patricia Kaminski, associate professor of psychology at the University of North Texas.[4] This often becomes a problem with collegiate scholarship athletes, who are under significant pressure to perform well both academically and athletically to keep their scholarships. The National Eating Disorder Information Centre (NEDIC) in Canada defines four types of eating disorders: anorexia nervosa, anorexia athletica, bulimia nervosa, and disordered eating. Another vital syndrome is the female athlete triad, and exercise bulimia has recently been recognized. Eating disorders have the highest death rate of any psychiatric illness. At the University of Michigan, an estimated 25 to 31 percent of students engage in disordered eating behaviors.[5]

GENETICS, FAMILY DYNAMICS, AND EATING DISORDERS

Competitiveness and sports-related pressures aren't the only reasons female athletes can develop eating disorders. Recent studies, in fact, have indicated that genetics and family dynamics can play an important role in whether people are more or less susceptible to engaging in disordered eating behaviors.

Genetics

In a 2013 *Time* magazine article, experts confirmed what they have long suspected: genetic factors probably contribute to problems with appetite and feelings of fullness, issues that put some female athletes more at risk than others for disordered eating and eating disorders. Researchers at the University of Iowa and University of Texas Southwestern Medical Center have discovered two different gene mutations that may point to families at higher risk for eating disorders. They studied two families with multiple eating-disordered family members across three and four generations, and in both families studied, they discovered rare genetic mutations that they believe actually increase the risk of eating disorders. It's been noted for years that eating disorders tend to run in families; now, it seems, it's possible to identify the reason for this trend using genetics.

A 2010 study through the University of California, San Diego, looked at the genes of two thousand women who had eating disorders compared with women who had never had eating disorders, using brain imaging (fMRIs) to study the brain activity of the two groups. The study found that no single genes create eating disorders; rather anorexics and bulimics have specific personality traits that stand out, including a high degree of anxiety, self-consciousness, obsessive thinking, and perfectionism. A striking finding from this study suggests that anxiety plays a crucial role in one's risk of developing an eating disorder.[6]

Family Dynamics

Family dynamics play an important role in body image and eating issues. In an article about the family structure of eating disorders, Whitney Spannuth (an Olympic cross-country runner who has suffered from eating disorders herself) points to four different aspects of functioning that may be involved in the family of an anorexic female: (1) family members are overly involved in each other's lives, (2) family members (especially parents) are overly controlling or overprotective, (3) parents are rigid and invested in situations and behaviors staying the way they are (especially when adolescents are pushing for more independence), and (4) family members exhibit discomfort with any type of conflict and an inability to deal with and resolve conflict. These inflexible family dynamics may increase a female athlete's propensity for developing some form of disordered eating or an actual eating disorder. Other risk factors include sexual or physical abuse or a mother who engages in disordered eating or has an eating disorder (these moms often serve irregular meals and junk food and focus constantly on their daughter's weight from a young age).

In some situations a family becomes rigid, intrusive, and enmeshed in direct response to the development of a child's eating disorder. When this occurs, the eating-disordered athlete is the family's focus. No one is talking about or even acknowledging the problem, but everyone is changing his or her behavior in order to accommodate that individual's needs and often resenting the individual for it. When this is the case, it is particularly important that the family be included in the child's treatment.

DISORDERED EATING

"Disordered eating" is a term that covers the gamut of eating problems. The mildest form of disordered eating is characterized by low-level and/ or occasional abnormal eating behaviors. Disordered eating may have a negative effect on a person's emotional, physical, and social well-being but not to the extremes that full-blown eating disorders do. Disordered eating includes such behaviors as eliminating food groups and meals, comparing your eating habits to others', basing your self-worth on how much food you've eaten, feeling guilty about eating certain foods, excessive weighing, calorie counting, constant dieting, overexercising to make up for a big meal the night before, and avoiding thinking about physical hunger and your need to feel full.

Years ago, I met with a young swimmer, Laura, and her mother. When it became clear that the mother's rigidity was contributing to the girl's eating problems (which, in turn, were affecting her swimming performances), the mother stopped coming to sessions with her daughter. This was helpful during our sessions, because Laura could speak more freely without her mother there, but unfortunately the family's rigidity in her day-to-day life reinforced some of the behaviors that we worked on changing. Her swimming performance did improve as she got a better handle on her disordered eating, but even that didn't seem to be enough for her mom, who demanded perfection, which is a big part of why Laura began to engage in disordered eating in the first place.

EATING DISORDERS

Female athletes with eating disorders shift to extreme behaviors with regard to food, often severely starving themselves. The hallmarks of anorexia and bulimia are denial and preoccupation with food and weight. Individuals with anorexia and bulimia tend to be high achievers, very competitive, obsessive about comparing themselves to others, negative, and dying for acceptance. They strive for perfection but never accept their efforts as good enough, and they often end up feeling emotionally isolated. Female athletes with eating disorders tend to look at food not as the necessary nutrition to keep their bodies healthy but rather as a way to exert control.

Years ago, a female cross-country runner from a college in my area was referred to me by her father. Upon further assessment, Lucy divulged that her entire team had eating issues, including anorexia, bulimia, and anorexia-bulimia; they were all either starving themselves, vomiting after meals, or both. When I offered to speak with her team, she indicated that the coach encouraged her and her team members to be this way, emphasizing to them the importance of doing whatever it took to win, including staying thin and eating very little. At the time, this was quite shocking to me; soon, though, I discovered that this was a common practice, especially among male coaches.

Laura's story is just one of many cases I've seen in which a coach or family member encouraged rather than discouraged improper eating and engaging in eating disorders. This illustrates how influential the attitudes of the people surrounding female athletes (especially people in positions of authority) can be. There are five types of eating disorders relevant to athletes: anorexia nervosa, anorexia athletica, bulimia nervosa, exercise bulimia, and the female athlete triad. We'll go into detail about each of them here.

Anorexia Nervosa

Anorexia nervosa, briefly described, involves self-starvation, a severely distorted body image, fear of gaining weight, a need for control, and obsessive thinking about the body and food. Individuals with this disorder obsess about food and develop a "starvation" state of mind. They are 15 percent or more below ideal body weight and often think they are fat, despite the fact that they're severely underweight. They often have underlying psychological issues, such as depression and anxiety. According to researcher Dr. Walter Kaye, "Anorexia nervosa has the highest rate of death of any psychiatric illness."[8]

I briefly worked one summer with a female collegiate runner who appeared healthy and fit but kept remarking that she needed to lose weight. She had originally been referred to me for issues of depression, but to me it seemed that her issues went beyond depression: she was entrenched in anorexic thinking and faced continual problems with stress fractures, two big warning signs that her parents didn't appear to be seeing. She did not want me to express any of my concerns to her parents or anyone else, and therefore I couldn't since she was twenty-one and considered an adult. Her college athletic team did seem to be addressing the problem, but even so, she remained in total denial.

Distinct physical and emotional/behavioral symptoms accompany anorexia, some of which we've covered already. Additional symptoms include the following.

Physical symptoms:

- Excessive weight loss
- Fatigue
- Extremely thin appearance (often with ribs showing)
- Dizziness or fainting
- Insomnia
- Soft, downy hair covering the body
- Intolerance of cold
- Irregular heart rhythms
- Swelling of arms or legs
- Abnormal blood counts
- Constipation
- Brittle nails
- Low blood pressure

- Pasty skin
- Hair loss or thinning

Emotional/behavioral symptoms:

- Denial of hunger
- Restricted food intake
- Lying about food intake
- Fear of weight gain
- Food rituals
- Constant criticism of appearance
- Distorted sense of body image
- Anxiety
- Depression
- Anger
- Irritability

Hollie Avil, a 2008 British Olympian, gave up her triathlon spot for the 2012 games when it came out that her shin stress fractures were due to her struggle with anorexia. For Avil, it all began at the end of a race in 2006, when a coach (not hers) said, "You'll need to start thinking about your weight if you want to run quick, Hollie." This one comment caused Avil to start obsessing about food. She did seek help from a psychologist and nutritionist, a step that allowed her to get a handle on her disorder for two years, but she relapsed in 2010. When she faced her disorder again in 2011 and sought treatment a second time, she was additionally diagnosed with depression. In May 2012, at the age of twenty-three, after already having been a double world champion, a national champion, and ranked number one in the world, Avil decided to end her career.[9]

KD, a Marin County trainer, says she struggled with anorexia when she was in high school and college. An only child, she grew up with a verbally abusive father who constantly called her "pig." She became a perfectionist and dedicated dancer (she admired her dance teacher, who had her students weigh themselves once a week and then posted their weight on the wall of the dance studio for everyone to see). This public display is never a good idea to practice with girls. In high school, KD drastically reduced how much she ate, limiting herself to a starvation diet. At night, alone in her room, she would be so hungry that she would cry herself to sleep. She struggled with constant sickness, missed a lot of school, and was significantly underweight during her junior year. At her lowest point, early in her senior year, KD decided to quit dancing and began to allow herself larger portions. Having enough energy to keep up her studies made her senior year in high school much easier.

KD's first two years of college were a little shaky, and in her last two years, her anorexia became more pronounced; she even lost a boyfriend due to her eating disorder. At one point, a family member whom she admired warned her that her disorder could affect her ability to have children—something she wanted badly. Finally, KD began to permit herself to eat more (though she was still controlling about her food intake), and she took the courageous step of going to therapy for additional assistance. When she met the man who would eventually become her husband and he also expressed concern about her eating disorder, she was inspired to work even harder to unwind her tight food controls. "I began to allow more foods and experiment with what would happen if I added certain foods back into my diet," KD explains. "I did it ever so slowly, loosening my food rules, and saw that I didn't balloon up in weight as I thought would happen. I remember one of my rules was one tablespoon of peanut butter a week and one ounce of cheese a week. Now I eat them every day. . . . I still have some food rules, but they're geared more around health than weight and calories." Today, KD, a nutritionist, runs, eats nutritionally, and enjoys life with her husband and four children.

Anorexia Athletica

Although there is no official diagnosis, NEDIC recognizes another type of anorexia besides anorexia nervosa: anorexia athletica. This condition involves compulsive exercising in an effort to "control your body." For those who suffer from anorexia athletica, or exercise addiction, this compulsive exercising is the only way to feel power and experience self-worth. These individuals are overly obsessed with weight and dieting, are never satisfied with their outcomes in athletic events, and never take rest days (for fear of losing control and gaining weight). One caveat: Olympic or pro athletes display some of these behaviors in their training; the difference is that they also build in rest times so they don't overtax their bodies.

Bulimia Nervosa

The main characteristic of bulimia nervosa is engaging in frequent bouts of binge eating and purging. Immediately after binging, bulimics make themselves throw up; use laxatives, enemas, diuretics, or diet pills; or fast. A bulimic can consume as many as three to five thousand calories in little more than an hour and as many as twenty thousand calories in eight hours when binging. Like anorexics, however, these individuals have an excessive fear of gaining weight, which is why they follow each binge with a purge.

Bulimics often appear to have a normal weight, or their weight may fluctuate up and down significantly. Bulimics, like anorexics, try to keep their problem secret—hiding their behavior from friends and family, sneaking off to the bathroom after a meal or waiting until a public bathroom is cleared out in order to purge. The purging itself may be representative of their need for control or punishment. More often than not, bulimics will generally refuse help until some sort of physical, psychological, or sports-related crisis is reached.

Other physical and emotional symptoms of bulimia (some of which are crossovers from anorexia) include the following.

Physical symptoms:

- Dry or loose skin
- Broken blood vessels in the eyes
- Smell of vomit
- Mouth problems (decaying teeth or sores)
- Scars or calluses on knuckles or hands
- Kidney failure
- Lightheadedness, loss of balance, or fainting
- Irregular heartbeats and palpitations
- Frequent weight changes

Emotional/behavioral symptoms:

- Sneaking or hiding food
- Noticeable preoccupation with body image or weight
- Feelings of shame and humiliation
- Avoidance of eating in public or with others
- Poor self-esteem

- Mood swings
- Anxiety or depression

Kimiko Hirai Soldati, a 2004 Olympic diver, first started participating in gymnastics in high school, where she had a coach who placed a lot of emphasis on keeping her weight low. When Soldati started diving, her coach for that sport told her whole team, "Don't get fat." These directions clearly sent the message, "Do whatever it takes to stay thin, or you'll be a failure in gymnastics and diving." Soldati began her binging and purging while still in high school. At first she only purged once in a while, when panicked about having eaten too much. In college, however, her binging and purging became so bad that her roommate finally confronted her. Luckily, Soldati was willing to get help; she was sick and tired of being sick and tired. She attended an eating disorders program at a nearby hospital, where she learned about healthy versus unhealthy eating and discovered that she was not alone. After dealing with her bulimia, she went on to be named "US Diver of the Year" in 2001 and 2002 and eventually to qualify for the 2004 Olympic team. She's given back by speaking in public about eating disorders, sharing her own story to help others.

Exercise Bulimia

In exercise bulimia, athletes obsess about exercising; they binge on food, then purge through excessive exercise. Compulsive overtraining or exercising relieves these athletes of the guilt they feel for eating and allows them to act on the belief that they need to lose weight. Female athletes suffering from exercise bulimia usually maintain a normal weight, which makes their disorder more difficult to identify. Their excessive workouts, however, can be so intense that they create a whole myriad of medical, mental, sports-related, and social problems.

The physical effects of exercise bulimia generally show up as fatigue or exhaustion, reproductive problems, dehydration, arthritis, cardiovascular difficulties, stress fractures due to osteoporosis, and poor performance in competition. Again, this can be a rather difficult form of eating disorder to identify, especially in athletes with demanding training programs. The following behaviors, however, are distinct signs of exercise bulimia:

- Exercise or training that takes priority over everything
- Feelings of guilt when unable to stick with a training or exercise routine
- Refusal to eat if unable to exercise
- Insistence on exercising or training even when injured or sick
- Pronounced feelings of anxiety if a workout day is missed
- Exercising or training's becoming the main source of control in the individual's life

Female Athlete Triad

The most complicated eating disorder suffered by athletic girls and women is the female athlete triad, which consists of three conditions: eating disorders, amenorrhea, and osteoporosis. The eating disorders involved in the female athlete triad are usually anorexia, anorexia-bulimia, or bulimia. These serious eating disorders create problems with energy (because of a lack of food intake), starvation thinking and eating, and, in the case of bulimia, binging and purging. These abnormal eating habits prevent individuals from receiving adequate nutrition.

Amenorrhea is the absence of menstrual periods, a condition that can lead to hormone imbalances and lower estrogen levels. A combination of factors contributes to amenorrhea, including inadequate nutrition, high energy demands, stress, and a low body mass index. Lowered estrogen levels from lack of menstruation, meanwhile, can contribute to bone loss and lack of concentration.

There are two types of amenorrhea: primary and secondary. In primary amenorrhea, a young female athlete has not gotten her first menstrual period by age fifteen. In secondary amenorrhea, the athlete misses three consecutive periods for no apparent reason. A female athlete with menstrual problems needs to be evaluated by a physician, since there are a number of reasons for an individual to miss her periods.

The third component of female athlete triad, osteoporosis, is a condition in which a female athlete has low bone density, putting her at risk for bone fractures. This kind of bone loss, which occurs due to a lack of calcium and low estrogen levels, reduces bone mass and strength, causing the bones to become more brittle. When their bones become brittle, female athletes are more likely to suffer shin fractures or stress fractures in the foot, injuries that tend to heal slower in athletes with osteoporosis.

This occurs more commonly in connection with anorexia than with bulimia.

IDENTIFYING AND TREATING EATING DISORDERS

Female athletes prone to the eating disorders discussed in this chapter are put at greater risk by the pressure exerted by the relationships surrounding them, including with parents, coaches, and the media. High school students vying to get college scholarships and college students trying to perform well in order to maintain the scholarships they've been awarded are at greater risk as well, as are young women experiencing periods of transition, such as from high school to college. High-risk young women may also struggle with low self-worth, depression, or anxiety.

Unfortunately, despite how prevalent they are among female athletes, eating disorders are difficult to identify. Even when they are identified, it's almost always a struggle to get an eating-disordered athlete to recognize her problem and accept appropriate assistance; denial is a cornerstone of eating disorders. Identification therefore comes mainly through coaches, teammates, friends, and family members rather than from the athletes themselves. The National Collegiate Athletic Association has written a comprehensive coach's handbook on eating disorders, *Managing the Female Athlete Triad*, which can be found online as a free PDF. Every coach should have a copy (and it wouldn't hurt for parents to have one as well).

Learning to identify the signs and symptoms of eating disorders is important for those who work with female athletes. When an eating disorder is identified in a female athlete, the most effective treatment plan is usually for her to see a licensed therapist trained in sports psychology, a sports-oriented nutritionist, and medical personnel to provide guidance tailored to her needs. For an eating-disordered individual who's kept a lot of things secret, working on establishing trust should be the primary goal.

Once that trust is established, when it seems useful and appropriate, it can also be very important for a psychologist to communicate with the athlete's coaches. This collaborative style is the most useful for getting an athlete all the help she needs and will help her to look more at the whole picture rather than just the details (which is especially vital when it comes to nutrition).

Other resources for female athletes suffering from eating disorders include support groups, family therapy, nutritional counseling, and possible medications for depression and anxiety disorders. If more serious medical or psychological problems develop, in- and outpatient clinics and hospital programs may be necessary. Throughout all of this, it's important that a female athlete's loved ones, teammates, and coaches offer the help, reassurance, and support she needs. According to Dr. Haleh Kashani, director since 2000 of the eating disorders program at Kaiser Permanente in San Rafael, California, the main goal during recovery is for the eating-disordered athlete to change her relationship with herself, to feel self-compassion, and, ultimately, to accept herself just as she is.

CHANGING OUR PERSPECTIVE

Though much has improved for women in general since the passage of Title IX, body image remains a difficult topic for many female athletes today, and until the media quits focusing on the "Ten Hottest Women in Sports" and starts focusing on the actual accomplishments of female athletes, it will continue to be a difficult subject. As long as we focus only on the 2 percent of women who meet the media's ridiculous beauty standards, body image dissatisfaction will continue to run rampant, and eating disorders will continue to grow in number. Ultimately, though, regardless of our society's skewed vision of what an "ideal" athlete should look like, the fact remains that female athletes who train thoughtfully, eat nutritionally, get plenty of rest, and socialize with their teammates and competitors (not female athletes who starve and overwork themselves) are more likely not only to have a positive body image but to perform better in their sport.

TEN MENTAL STRATEGIES FOR MAINTAINING A POSITIVE BODY IMAGE

1. Focus on positive thoughts about your body.
2. Keep a journal about your feelings.
3. Keep active with friends, especially fellow athletes.

4. Maintain a healthy relationship with food. Consider consulting a sports nutritionist.
5. Maintain a routine for your workouts and build your efforts in time, aided by others.
6. Focus on how your clothes fit rather than on your weight or the size you wear.
7. Wear clothes you feel comfortable and happy in.
8. Let go of perfection.
9. Learn to accept yourself and your body type.
10. Learn to be proud of your body.

7

TEAM SPIRIT

Practicing Collaboration and Camaraderie

The energy of hundreds of female athletes together is powerful. In April 2010, on the first night of the Luna Chix Summit in Berkeley, California, this power was in evidence as scores of female cyclists, mountain bikers, runners, and triathletes gathered together in celebration of a common cause: supporting each other through sports. That night, pro and amateur female athletes alike mingled, exchanged jokes, and talked about the meaning of sports in their lives.

Like the Luna Chix women, girls and women in every walk of life are buoyed by peer connections. Unlike male athletes, who tend to form hierarchies on their teams, female athletes tend to relate to their team members as friends they can talk about their personal lives with and confide in. As Coach Ken Grace once explained, girls in sports form a circle, wanting to connect, while boys form a ladder, each wanting to kick the last guy off.

Team spirit grows from positive team dynamics and consists of collaboration, cooperation, community, loyalty, and solidarity. Team spirit is created by enthusiastic attitudes about playing with other team members. Each player's positive attitude is supportive of the team's goals and purpose, which are best set up by inclusion of the whole team's input. This is a way to encourage all the team members to commit to the team's mission. As a high school basketball player once said to me, team spirit means "playing for everyone on the team." Basically, a bonded team with spirit turns in good performances. Teams whose members talk to each other, express enthusiasm for their sport, work hard, value cooperation, show dedication, and encourage each other are far more likely to succeed. As Anni M., a young woman who played soccer throughout high school and college, wrote in a blog post about team spirit, "When you care more about your team's success than your own, individual agendas fade into the background. . . . Teams provide a mini-community, a social network that depends on every member's hard work."[1]

These sporting skills easily extend into life after sports. Hopefully, with your female teammates, you strive to become a team player through shared goals for the team. Avigiel "Ace" Cohen, a senior female basketball player and captain at the University of California, Berkeley, reflected on the 2012–2013 season as the best of her life. That year, the team beat Stanford at their house, became Pac10 Champions, and constantly exposed themselves to the media when they reached the Final Four. These were all first-time events in the forty-year history of the Berkeley women's basketball team. The teammates didn't want to separate at the end of the season and were willing to do anything for each other. Ace is still in touch with the four departing seniors despite the distances separating them. Mikayla Lyles, a senior and another team captain, felt like she learned to better connect with others and that this connection meant more for the team as a whole. "I became the encourager and supporter. My role was to provide support with a 100% commitment, helping others be better at every game, encouraging teammates to learn from the coach, and do whatever else was needed."

A remarkable example of a team with plenty of team spirit is the 1996 Atlanta Olympics women's soccer team and the 1999 World Championship team (thirteen of whose sixteen players had also been on the 1996 Olympic team). Women's soccer was included in the Olympics for the first time in 1996, and the team was tight and well led by head coach Tony DiCicco, whose positive team-building approaches worked well for female athletes. He brought a sports psychologist, Dr. Colleen Hacker, aboard to work on his players' mental skills and to facilitate team bonding. Afterward, many of the players attributed at least part of their success to the team's positive dynamics. Remarkably, the final 1996 match drew the largest crowd ever to gather for a women's sporting event at that time. The turnout was 76,481 fans who watched as the United States held off China to win the gold. As Tiffeny Milbrett scored the winning goal with a series of great shots by teammates, a roar went up from the US crowd. The entire international soccer community had high praise for the outstanding US women's team and the US victory. Mia Hamm reflects, "To me, one of the reasons we were successful was that we respected and cared about the game and felt the same way about each other. . . . [My teammates] always understood there was a greater purpose. That the opportunity to play was extremely special, and let's try to make sure as many young girls have that opportunity." Ultimately, this focus on positivity and collaboration helped the team bring home the gold.

TEAM SPIRIT ESSENTIALS

In women's sports, both individual and group, cooperation, spoken communication, and empathy are vital. This means that teams shouldn't be allowed to get too cliquey; rather, they should be encouraged to form a circle, a group in which they can connect equally with one another on an intimate (emotional) level and add or release players as needed. This approach builds a foundation that allows the members of a team to work together successfully. As Michael Jordan once said, "Talent wins games and teamwork and intelligence win championships."

The most successful female sports teams have a clear vision or goal. Team spirit blossoms most when players are able to rally around a common purpose. This is important for girls because they need to like the girls they play with. Many long-term friendships among older athletes stem from membership on high school and college teams. I worked with a young (thirty-year-old) female police officer, Katy, whose best friends were still the women from her college field hockey team. They talked frequently and organized get-togethers throughout the year despite living in different spots around the United States. When they played together, the team had loads of fun on and off the field, according to Katy.

FEMALE ATHLETES IN INDIVIDUAL SPORTS

Even in individual sports, bonding is an important piece of the puzzle. At the 2012 London Olympics, we watched many of the top female swimmers cheer and support each other during individual events. The camaraderie their mutual support created meant that team spirit was already present when it came time for the relays, which require a more collaborative effort.

Female athletes perform their best when they come together in conditions where they perform together in a spirit of teamwork. This is largely because female relationships have an emotional component that causes women to relate to others in a different way than males do. Even in sports where you compete alone, you can always train with fellow teammates, creating an opportunity for the sharing and daring that will allow you to help each other improve. Pushing your fellow athletes, and getting pushed by them, in a collaborative and bonding way can help you all compete even harder and better.

Cross-country is largely thought of as an individual sport, but with the proper guidance, teammates can exhibit incredible team spirit. When I started working with the City College of San Francisco cross-country team, I saw tremendous cooperation and collaboration in the way the girls related to one another. Their upbeat tone was evident. Each one felt known as an individual and yet that she formed part of a unified team. Each team member had individual goals, as did the team as a whole. The coach placed a lot of emphasis on bonding and fun: the team had an annual retreat at Lake Tahoe, and in addition to the daily runs, the girls spent lots of time hanging out and getting to know each other. Coach Ken and I did seminars for the team members aimed at building team spirit. Fun was also an important element in these retreats.

I was brought in to discover any unknown issues and to help the girls push past them to improve their performances even further. The general goal for each girl depended on where she ranked in the team's running times. The primary goal was for each team member to improve her individual performance to the best of her ability. After my first talk, one member of the team, Susan, surprised herself, her team members, and her coach by dramatically reducing her time for the two mile. When I first came to the team, her best time was 14.5 minutes; by the end of the season, it was 12 minutes. Susan wasn't the only one who experienced such a huge improvement, either. It seemed that giving the young women on the team permission to push beyond their own limits (and encouraging them to support each other as they did so) provided the impetus some of them needed to flourish. The teammates were collaboratively competitive with each other, cheering the other girls who finished behind them. Annually, they would go to a retreat at another coaches' home in Lake Tahoe. There were always daily runs but lots of hanging out and getting to know each other.

FEMALE ATHLETES IN TEAM SPORTS

In team sports, team spirit is essential to positive performance and outcomes. The more consistent the team bonding and cooperation, the more likely team members are to work positively together toward success. As basketball coach Phil Jackson has emphasized, "The strength of the team is each individual member. The strength of each member is the team." This can be true for both female and male athletes, but it is especially essential for female athletes.

If you've ever observed young athletes interacting on their own, you've probably noticed the difference between the girls and the boys. Upon entering a gym, girls and women are more easily distracted by the external stimuli around them. Males can play even if angry at another team member, whereas females can find it more difficult to put aside the personal stuff. Young female athletes will most likely get in a circle and pass the ball around. Young male athletes, in contrast, are more likely to take to the court immediately and play a competitive game. Take long-time volleyball coach Bill Neville's observation of what happened at the 1990 Olympic Sports Festival: "The women's teams spent most of their practice time on technique and positioning drills, while the men's teams spent most of their practice time in competitive, game-like drills."[2] In other words, there was a noticeable difference in the way the male and female volleyball players practiced.

Mary McLain, a Marin County attorney, describes herself as a team player with a positive attitude, an ability to reach goals and objectives, and great personal drive and stamina. Her co-captain on her women's tennis team, Tracy McCullough, describes herself as perseverant, disciplined, and fun. When their team had a chance to move up to A1 a few years back, the co-captains decided to hold their team back in order to combine forces with another team that was struggling and about to move down. The next year, they set up active communication channels with the newly combined team, established team goals, and began holding weekly team practices. By the end of the year, they had won the trophy for the A2 level and were moving up to play in the A1 level, and according to Mary and Tracy, they were in a stronger place than they had been the year prior. In other words, these two female teams accomplished more by joining together than they would have been able to accomplish alone.

Not only is this amateur tennis team strong in competition, but its members' bonds are strong off the court. When Mary's daughter had cancer, the entire team provided support for the family—visiting frequently and supplying home-cooked meals. Mary says she felt completely cared for by all her teammates during that time, and their strengthened rapport has only improved their performances on the court even further.

THE FIVE STAGES OF TEAM DYNAMICS

There are many ways to look at group or team dynamics for females. We know that communication for girls and women is best done through talking and the written word (texts and e-mails, for example). Given what we know about female athletes' strengths, the other important qualities to consider when looking at their team dynamics include emotional connections with those around them, one-on-one friendships, empathy and intuition, peer-group camaraderie and cooperation, and the inclusion of fun in their training and competitions.

American psychologist Bruce Tuckman (1965, 1977) created a five-stage model for groups that can easily be adapted to female athletic teams with the addition of using a backward/forward and circular style. Simply put, the stages are forming, storming, norming, performing, and adjourning.

Forming

In the forming stage, the formal (coach) and less formal (players) leaders help other players on a team to develop confidence and trust in one another and to establish regular communication channels. This is the critical time when players are getting to know one another and form into a group. During this stage, common goals and objectives for the team should be discussed and determined, and clear and concise instructions about training and competitions should be presented. Female athletes, in particular, will benefit from two primary considerations during this time:

(1) being reassured that they are cared about, and (2) receiving thorough explanations about the complexity of skills they will be expected to execute. All female teams are more likely to accept a new player if they like her. The team's motivation is directly impacted by the tone and sensitivity of the coach and players; if there is more negative than positive feedback, the tone of the group will be influenced in that direction. Since female athletes respond better to being told what they should do rather than what they shouldn't do, taking a more positive approach is most helpful during this and every other stage.

Storming

In the storming stage, team members argue about the structure of the team, which makes for conflicts that may affect the team's performance. Inconsistency, lack of cohesion, resentment, frustration, unspoken agendas, and judgments can all come into play at this time, as might women's tendency to work toward a quick resolution. Most teammates will look to the formal and informal leaders of the team for guidance and structure to resolve the conflict. With teens especially, it's important that coaches identify and work on connecting with informal leaders.

I saw a perfect example of the storming stage while working with a newly established girls' basketball team. Susan, one of the older members of the team, was often critical of the younger players, and she delivered her criticisms in an unhelpful manner. After we worked together for a while, the younger players confronted Susan. Putting the issue out in the open like this cleared the air for all grievances to be discussed and resolved and eventually contributed to the group becoming more cohesive. Ultimately, the best way to move through the storming stage with success is to establish guidelines that clarify each player's role and responsibility.

Norming

In the norming stage, the team cooperatively comes together. The players begin to listen to and support each other, show an appreciation for each other's strengths, and accept each other's weaknesses, and the flow of the team really is seen. This is when a team becomes a cohesive unit and attains more peak performances.

A prime example of a team that reached the norming stage is the 2012–2013 Berkeley women's basketball team. One very talented player on the team, Avigiel "Ace" Cohen, a former Israeli national team member, suffered a severe, career-ending injury in her first year of play. Instead of letting her go, however, the team recognized her superior leadership skills and decided to make her one of the captains. That act is just one example of the many ways that year's team members displayed respect and admiration for one another, according to the two senior players interviewed. "The team members were willing do anything for each other, and considered each other sisters," said Ace. This is the kind of bonding and positivity found in the norming stage.

Performing

In the performing stage, a collaborative and cohesive team has formed. The leaders' and players' hard work has paid off, and the team is achieving its goals. Here, the biological strengths of females come into play. The team members are openly, verbally communicative, show empathy for one another, act collaboratively, express confidence, and win games. The now interdependent group is able to adjust its play according to the strengths and weaknesses of its players and those on other teams.

Not all teams will reach this stage, but Berkeley's 2012–2013 team did. Another team member, Mikayla Lyles, says all the team's members were motivated and played like a cohesive unit that year. Mikayla describes their win over Stanford (in Stanford's house, no less) as "an incredible accomplishment" for the team. "It wasn't necessarily breaking [Stanford's] eighty-one-game winning streak," she says. "It was that we did it as a team. . . . We came off a loss and made it happen."

This stage is difficult for any team to reach, but it is well worth striving for. As Ace and Mikayla said, playing with a team that has reached the performing level is "magical."

Adjourning

Adjourning, the last of the five stages, has to do with the shifting of a team or group of players when they experience significant changes, for instance at the end of a season. Some players may be saying good-bye (either forever or temporarily), and the team readies itself for change.

Berkeley's 2012–2013 women's basketball team struggled with this stage. After such a good run together, the teammates simply didn't want to separate. Unfortunately, as college players, they had no choice in the matter: four of their starters, including their best player, Talia Caldwell, were graduating seniors. All the women who left considered each other sisters, including Ace, who says she's still in touch with three of them. Ace describes 2013 as the best year of her life—in large part due to her team's dynamics and successes. This team of female athletes constantly believed in themselves and thoroughly trusted each other on and off the court.

ACHIEVING SUCCESS AT ANY STAGE

For a team to gel and work through the five stages of development discussed above, it's helpful to keep the following in mind:

- Female athletes work best in a circle, rotating responsibilities and roles.
- The goals of the team should be expressed clearly and concisely.
- In order for the team to work collaboratively, it's essential to establish ground rules early on.
- Conflict is normal and inevitable; find positive ways to resolve issues that arise.
- It's essential that leaders and players listen to each other.
- Doing wrap-up sessions after training and games keeps communication open.
- Encouraging each player's participation builds team cohesion.

THE BUILDING BLOCKS OF TEAM SPIRIT

Team spirit was present in spades in the 1980 US Olympic women's fencing team. Stacey Johnson, who was on the team (and who is now a former Executive Olympic Committee member and former president of the Olympic Fencing Committee), says she has always valued having a "circle of wise women in her life," and her team that year provided exactly that. Despite having an unsupportive mother, Stacey bonded closely with Gay D'Asaro, who was her teammate on the 1980 Olympic team, and with a third fencer, Vinnie Bradford, whom they fenced with on some international teams and who participated in the 1984 Olympics. Together, they were "warrior sisters," according to Stacey. "The key to our excellence was our innovation in the mental, spiritual, and psychological realms." They all ended up in the Fencing Hall of Fame, and thirty-some years later, they are still best friends.

Stacey Johnson expresses her perspective on team spirit in this way:

> What I believe about those teams, and even the teams I serve on today in higher education, is that there are certain principles that assist in building strong leadership and collaboration in teams. Teams need to have a shared dream or vision; they need to support one another in the quest of those dreams; they need teams to know and understand that they have the power to change previously negative outcomes through work and support of each other; they need to persevere and not give up; they need to look for mentors and coaches who can help them achieve their dreams and vision; they need to know that if they lead to serve the others on the team, things usually work out better; they should seek to make things better for others and pay it forward to the next group following them; and finally, their individual members need to listen and reflect on their own inner voice and knowingness, particularly when making decisions . . . and then go for it!

Building on Stacey's words, the following are some of the most vital building blocks of team spirit.

Strong Leadership

Once the captains of a team, the formal leaders, engage with teammates and build positive connections, the foundation and structure of the group are being created. Positive leadership is particularly important for female athletes. Captains Ace Cohen and Mikayla Lyles of the Berkeley women's basketball team emphasize how important their desire to help and encourage their teammates was. Mikayla talked about four essential approaches that helped her as one of the team's captains: (1) making a solid commitment to everything related to the team, (2) helping her teammates improve, (3) attending every practice and game, and (4) being open to learning from the coaches.

In order for team spirit to truly thrive, a team's leaders and players must also listen and talk to one another. Since women's main communication method is talking, engaging female athletes in active group discussions is a useful tool for coaches and captains. Taking the time to speak to players in a constructive way (rather than yelling negative criticisms at them) is helpful as well. Strong, positive connections can enhance the entire athletic experience for all athletes, especially female athletes.

Balancing Collaboration with Competition

Team spirit is often affected by female athletes' conflicting desires to both "tend and befriend" and compete. Women's intrinsic need to please and get along with others can hinder their competitive nature and affect their athletic performance. As more time elapses since the passage of Title IX, we watch ever increasing numbers of young girls compete in sport. During the turbulence of their teen years, competitive young women often face peer and romantic pressure to stay in or get out of sports. The more athletic good friends teens have, the likelier they are to stay involved. By learning to have competitive girlfriends in youth, young women will hopefully learn to have competitive girlfriends as they age. In areas where youth sport is strong, athletic girls form friendships from an early age through high school into college. Their natural tendency toward cooperation[3] renders the drive to both collaborate and compete a dilemma. When approached the right way, however, collaboration and competition can successfully coexist in group or team training.

Over twenty years ago, when training for the Western States one-hundred-mile race, I ran every Tuesday afternoon for five months with a group of four other women: Martha, TJ, Hazel, and Debbie. We ran as hard as we could on those Tuesdays, pushing each other up and down the hills of Marin County, mainly on and around Mount Tamalpais. The group had two main goals: (1) to run the Cool Canyon Crawl 50K, and (2) to prepare Debbie and me for the Western States 100. In order to help one another, we shared our strengths with each other as much as possible. Debbie, Hazel, and Martha were great at burning the rocky trail downhill. My strength was flying on the uphills. TJ brought an element of competitiveness that encouraged us all to push ourselves harder. We worked together with a solid sense of support and total inclusiveness. When we all ran the Cool 50K, we finished close together, and through it all we enjoyed a sense of collaborative competition, remained positive, and had fun. In other words, we found a way to balance our desire to cooperate with our desire to compete.

Common Goals

Developing a common goal (besides "winning") is an excellent way to build team spirit. This common goal can have different meanings for different levels of teams. Remember, a team is not just about its star players; it's about working together and accomplishing more as a unit. So it's important to get the whole team together and to settle on a goal that makes sense based on the entire group's strengths and weaknesses and level of competition. If you're a coach, take the time to listen to everyone's input, and keep things fun and lively (particularly if you coach younger girls and teens). This is the time to listen to everyone and to flush out any potential conflicts between team members.

I worked with a national girls' mountain biking team (Whole Athlete) that had a fantastic goal: to be mentally present, perform to their best abilities, and have fun during races. As one of the young members, Victoria, put it, "My main mental tool is my attitude. As long as I love what I'm doing and am having fun, I'm doing my best. So much of racing is mental that being in the moment is everything and often the determining factor in a close race." When I talked to four of her teammates, Sofia, McKenzie, Josie, and Kate, they echoed the same philosophy. They were all on the same page, and that helped them compete at a higher level.

Keeping Sports Friendly

Girls, much more than boys, need to like their fellow teammates. When female teammates dislike each other, you are bound to see conflicts arise between them, no matter the sport. Take, for example, Jenny, a young softball pitcher I worked with who played high school and club softball. She complained that she and her best friend were the only players on their high school team who made any effort to express encouragement and team spirit during games. They yelled and cheered for other members, but the rest of the team just sat on the bench like a bunch of duds, according to Jenny, which frustrated her and made her not like them very much.

During her four years in high school, Jenny told me, her team usually made it to the playoffs, but they never went very far. Their coach often yelled negative epitaphs at the various players and embarrassed them in front of their peers. Their failure to bond resulted in a failure to succeed. Jenny contrasted this lack of team spirit with the closeness of the players on her club team: "All the players were great. We worked hard and had a lot of fun." Unsurprisingly, her club team had a much better record than her high school team.

Listening and Talking

Another important ingredient in team spirit is for leaders and players to listen and talk to each other. As our brains dictate, females' main tool for communicating is talking. In the teenage years, the amount of chatter that girls do lays the groundwork, as they become women. Engaging the athletes in active group discussions is a useful tool. Taking the time to speak to and not yell negative criticisms at players is a helpful approach. Good leaders both listen and talk to players. Females are particularly sensitive on this subject. Berkeley basketball captain Mikayla Lyles describes herself as expanding as a person and developing her skills to connect. By understanding giving, selflessness, and her intuitive sense of self, Mikayla watches connections enhance the entire athletic experience. These positive give-and-take relationships mean more for your team. Of the 2012–2013 team, she simply states, "There were incredible moments and winning against Stanford was one of them."

Having Fun

Fun plays an important role for female athletes, especially young ones. Teen girls participate in sports largely because it's fun; in fact, in one study, 76.3 percent of girls aged nine to twelve cited fun as their primary reason for being physically active.[4] Even over twenty years ago, girls expressed their desire to have fun while playing sport. Anyone working or living with girl athletes needs to discover ways to help the team's members enjoy their playing and competing. The cooperative nature of girls supports this notion of fun being a part of team spirit. As Nicole M. LaVoi, associate director of the Tucker Center for Research on Girls and Women in Sport, said in a 2013 *New York Times* piece, "We want our girls active and empowered. We don't want them demoralized and side-lined or inactive due to dropout. To keep them playing, parents and coaches must imbue sport with a spirit of fun."[5]

Team Cohesion

The idea of a shared identity for a team is especially appealing for female athletes, since girls and women place so much value on interpersonal connection. Team cohesion can only be achieved when players have a common meaning and purpose; without those things, your team will struggle.

In high school sports, looking toward girls who are informal leaders and encouraging them to motivate their teammates can attain team cohesion. Consider Selena, the high school basketball player I talked about in chapter 2 who yelled out that her level of motivation, on a scale of one to ten, was a "twenty-five." She was clearly an informal leader; her words inspired her team. These are the kinds of players who help their teams build a sense of a shared identity and move toward a common goal. On teams that achieve true cohesion, all the players feel a sense of inclusion, like they're part of a greater whole.

THE FINAL WORD ON TEAM SPIRIT

In training and competition, female athletes thrive on positive bonding and connections with their peers. Liking and enjoying their training partners is essential to female athletes. When they can call their teammates their sisters and best friends and feel they can depend on each and every one of them, they are bound to flourish. In creating team spirit, girls and women bond over the sports they love and improve their performance in ways they never could without their teammates' support. Female athletes train and compete to their best abilities (and have fun doing it!) when they have the power of team spirit behind them.

TEN MENTAL STRATEGIES FOR CREATING TEAM SPIRIT WITH FEMALE ATHLETES

1. Create team spirit through a common vision.
2. Remain positive; don't engage in negative criticisms of other players or yourself.
3. Listen and talk to other players.
4. Encourage your teammates, and cheer when they make good plays or do well.
5. Show your like and respect for your teammates.
6. Find ways to work collaboratively with your teammates.
7. Get to know each other and be inclusive.
8. Trust and use your intuitive sense.
9. Empower your teammates to succeed to the best of their abilities.
10. Find ways to have fun even while working hard.

8

COACHES ARE CORNERSTONES

When Dr. Bruce Ogilvie, a grandfather of sports psychology, researched young female athletes, he made the striking observation that the athletes responded best to coaches with a "relationship focus." Attending the Association of Applied Sports Psychology convention, I heard him make these remarks as far back as 1998. These relationship-oriented coaches worked hard to develop positive one-on-one relationships with their athletes and strove to build strong team camaraderie. The most successful girls reported feeling personally cared about.

As a sports psychologist working with young female athletes, I've found that the mental skills they develop through playing sports provides them with a basic foundation for life, and their coaches are the cornerstones of that skill development. Coaches play a vital role in the success of the individual athlete and the team as a whole; in fact, a coach's attitude sets the tone for the whole team and can make or break a season.

Old-school coaches who constantly yell negative epithets and don't pay attention to their players, except for the stars, have difficulty developing a cohesive team, because they create tension and resentment among the players, increase detrimental gossip, and generally set the female teams up for failure. They certainly do not build up their athletes' self-esteem and confidence. When I was in high school, my tennis coach didn't have a good word to say to anyone, especially the players who most needed help to improve. Her approach was to find an aspect of each player's game to criticize. By the end of my first season with her as my coach, her constant yelling and put-downs had not only failed to better my game but actually made it worse.

In contrast, there is no limit to what a coach who uses a positive, encouraging, and supportive style can achieve. Take Ken Grace, a California Community College Coach of the Year award winner with whom I personally worked for a couple of years. His manner pulled me in when I began doing track workouts with his group at Kezar Stadium in San Francisco to run a one-hundred-mile race. He taught me to be more open and willing to try new things, like using a heart rate monitor for feedback as an ultrarunner. With his help, I learned how to run harder by pushing up my heart rate (which, after using the monitor, I discovered was generally low) and drastically improved my race times. Ken's philosophy is to encourage the female runners he works with to "want to be active for the rest of their lives" (key word: "want"). He's all about positive reinforcement, and he gets results because of that.

As Ken's coaching approach illustrates, girls' brains want to work in a collaborative and cooperative manner. Developing female athletes' empathy, then, and encouraging their naturally intuitive sides is far more effective than trying to reprogram them to be something they're not. Make no mistake: girls are fully capable of doing the hard work required to excel. Expressing a positive attitude is not the same thing as coddling; rather, it is a very useful means of empowerment. A coach who captures a female team's attention with a supportive approach, who makes athletes feel listened to and valued, and who gets to know players on an individual level is a coach who knows how to play to female athletes' strengths.

A thread runs through the many interviews I've conducted with coaches who have shown themselves to be particularly effective with female athletes. Whether consciously or unconsciously, all of these coaches employ psychological strategies that help their athletes to thrive. They get to know their girls and help them bond in a circle. Particularly in team sports, they may have star players but work on team cohesion through encouraging the girls to appreciate one another's strengths and weaknesses. They all understand the importance of validating their athletes' feelings and building positive emotional connections on their teams, and they have figured out how to do these things while pushing their athletes to set goals and meet challenges. They have mastered the mental practices that help female athletes succeed in sports. And armed with the right tools, any coach out there can join their ranks.

THE COACH'S ROLE

Coaches play a variety of roles for female athletes. They can be mentors, teachers, gurus, or guides, and they can be anything from their players' best friend to their worst enemy. But the true role of the girls' coach is to help players build self-confidence and self-esteem. Remember, unlike boys, who compete to gain status, girls initially get involved in competitive sports primarily to have fun.[1] Being negative all the time is a sure way for a coach to take all the fun out of sports for girls (not to mention destroy their self-esteem), so it's important to cultivate a positive approach.

Positive practices to employ when working with a girls' team include the following:

- Establishing an upbeat approach
- Encouraging ongoing spoken communication with players by allowing (and initiating) conversations before and after games
- Holding periodic discussions with the team about technical and mental issues
- Encouraging initial competition by establishing goals and objectives for individuals and the team
- Providing constructive feedback
- Praising outstanding behavior and performance in private
- Talking to the whole group, not singling out individuals
- Explaining playing decisions to players
- Looking out for and calling attention to positive behavior from all the team members
- Encouraging competition in a positive but firm manner
- Asking the team for feedback after particularly hard games, events, or meets
- Providing inspirational words and phrases, maybe even a team slogan to be used at games

Practices and behaviors to avoid when working with female athletes include the following:

- Negative screaming and yelling
- Focusing only on the negatives

- Consistently singling out the most talented athlete on the team (other players will interpret this behavior as dismissive of their talents or participation)
- Employing the "just do it" approach (i.e., demanding better performances without explaining the strategy and technical issues behind them)
- Shaming and humiliating players who are struggling, especially in front of the whole team
- Commenting on athletes' weight or posting individual weights (this may set individuals up for disordered eating or an eating disorder)
- Criticizing the team heavily and not mentioning at least one positive after a particularly difficult game, event, or meet

THE NEW SCHOOL VERSUS THE OLD SCHOOL

There are two main types of coaches who work with female athletes today. For simplicity's sake, I call them "old-school" and "new-school" coaches. Old-school coaches generally use rough, strict, and aggressive approaches with their athletes. New-school coaches, in contrast, are aware and well informed; they recognize the unique needs of female athletes, work on group cohesion, and make efforts to coach them in a positive manner.

This is not to say that there are no old-school coaches out there who recognize the importance of intimate relationships for female athletes and support and encourage the girls they coach. These coaches may not always describe their coaching techniques as clearly as new-school coaches do, but their behaviors indicate that they have a greater awareness of their female athletes' needs. Take, for example, Mike Fanelli, former head coach of the US national running team and longtime coach of the Impalas, a nationally ranked women's racing team. Mike did most of his coaching prior to 2000, and his emphasis as a coach tended to be on setting goals and achieving results, but his athletes trusted him, and he understood that running races wasn't all about athletics. He once said that he preferred coaching women because they are more intimate and straightforward than men. In other words, Mike appreciated that his female athletes operated from a more emotional place and thrived on honest communication. He valued his athletes as individuals, and that's what made him such a good coach.

Tony DiCicco, coach of the gold-medal-winning 1996 US Olympic women's soccer team and the 1999 USA World Championship women's team, embodies many new-school coaching qualities; he still belongs in the old-school category, however, because he has publicly stated that girls are no different from boys, and his female athletes have felt compelled to confront him about his approach in the past (as when Mia Hamm told him, "Treat us like women but coach us like men"). Still, his book *Catch Them Being Good* makes it plain that DiCicco's style of coaching is perfectly suited to women and was key to his teams' wins in the Olympics and the Women's World Cup.

DiCicco's coaching philosophy contains a couple of critical key points regarding supporting women athletes. "Play hard, play fair, play to win, have fun," he writes. He goes on to say that "playing to win doesn't mean that winning is the end-all, but it's an important component of success. . . . You need to keep things in perspective and communicate that approach. . . . If you create an environment of fun . . . you will teach [athletes] discipline, team chemistry and confidence-building skills that will translate into other areas of their lives."[2]

DiCicco also acknowledges the importance of validating the feelings of his players (especially his female players). "Validating a person's feelings is something I learned while working with women," he says, and he reveals how he demonstrates empathy for his players through active listening, setting up one-on-one meetings with them, and admitting his mistakes. He even describes putting himself in his players' shoes when significant conflicts take place in order to better understand how they feel and work to resolve the situation. Essentially, Tony DiCicco is an example of an outstanding coach who is forward thinking in his approach to mentoring female athletes (even if he doesn't want to admit that male and female athletes are different from one another!).

Caren Horstmeyer was the coach of women's basketball teams at the University of California, Berkeley, for five years and at Santa Clara University for eleven. Currently, she runs Horstmeyer Hoops in the summer, which is an annual all-girls basketball camp for second to eighth graders in Marin County, California. She says her philosophy comes from a "work hard and challenge yourself" perspective, not a "buddy-buddy" perspective, but she brings many new-school approaches into her coaching nonetheless. She describes, for example, how she works on understanding each of her players on an individual level, providing extra attention on and off the court, and expressing empathy. She says that women tend, more than men, to be more social, care more about what other people think, and struggle with festering problems that they just can't let go of. Her main frustration as a coach has been the gossiping that her female players have engaged in behind each other's back. As a whole, though, she loves coaching girls and women, and she says the bottom line is this: "When the women respect your knowledge and feel you are behind them and actively show your support, they will work hard and strive for success."

Unfortunately, the rough, at times even abusive, type of old-school coaching is still very much alive. Recently, I was in a shoe store talking about my book to the store manager, when another woman, Beth, overheard me and joined the conversation, speaking about her daughter who plays on a high school volleyball team. Beth played volleyball when she was her daughter's age and at the collegiate level, and she loved every minute of it; she's concerned about her daughter, whose team is having problems with cohesion. The coach focuses primarily on the two star players, which is causing friction among the other players. Beth, who remembers how close she was to her teammates in high school and college, hates that her daughter is losing her love for the sport because of her coach's tactics, but she doesn't know what to do about it. I commented that the situation was not surprising given the approach of the coach.

A young softball player I worked with, Meghan, ran into the same situation with her high school coach. The coach favored a star pitcher on her team, to the point that even when the team was way ahead in a game, he would only occasionally bring Meghan in to pitch. When he did allow Meghan on the mound, he yelled at her the whole time. He had no interest in helping his players grow; he was only interested in winning. But as any good coach will tell you, pitting your players against one another and criticizing their every move is no way to create a winning team. And not giving everyone on the team a chance to perform can diminish players' confidence in their play. If they made the team, they deserve a chance to get in the game, even if they are not the top players.

PSYCHOLOGICAL CONSIDERATIONS WITH FEMALE ATHLETES

Ken Grace, the running coach I mentioned earlier, claims that coaching young women is much easier than coaching young men for the following reasons:

- Girls listen when it comes to coaching and teaching a new concept, whereas boys challenge.
- Girls generally underestimate their athletic and competitive ability; boys think they are better than they actually are.
- It is easier to create a team atmosphere with a group of young women; young men tend to quickly create a ranking system within the team, with each knowing his place on the ladder.

Whether or not girls are really easier to coach than boys, they are certainly different to coach, and it's essential for the coaches who work with them to understand the psychology behind those differences. Let's take a closer look at the mental considerations unique to female athletes.

Personal Connections

Female athletes do better when they feel like they're part of a team; however, in order to bond with their coaches and teammates, they need to feel like they're being seen as individuals. Relationships are paramount to females. That's why taking the time to establish an understanding of each individual player is a coach's first step toward building a solid female athletic team. Female athletes thrive when they connect on a personal level with their coaches and teammates.

In individual sports, of course, it is more difficult to create a team dynamic, because athletes are more likely to focus only on their own performance. Coaches can prevent players from isolating themselves by encouraging them to get to know each other and involving them in group activities; these things may sound unimportant in comparison to training, but they help build the type of relationships that females need and long for. Julia Violich, a former coach of the Whole Athlete girls' team and the current coach of the Bear Development racing team, always has personal relationships with all the girls on her teams. When she coached the Whole

Athlete girls' team, for example, Julia always rode with the girls, provided them with emotional support, and explained good nutrition to them; at their annual team retreat, she played music videos so they would dance together, sat up chatting with them at night, and even hennaed her and the girls' hair. Back in the Bay Area, Julia kept the girls' parents in the loop, communicated with the players and the parents through Facebook, and checked in with them about noncycling issues. She went out of her way to learn about her athletes, and it made her team stronger.

Open Communication and Positive Feedback

Since female athletes like to talk and ask questions, it's important that coaches make a concerted effort to listen to and communicate with them in an open and honest way. Being open and honest does not mean being harsh and highly critical, however; in fact, coaches should strive not to criticize their athletes, especially not in front of the team. No one likes to be dressed down in front of his or her peers, and girls and women are especially sensitive to this sort of treatment. If you have something to tell one of your athletes, you should take her aside, talk calmly, and try to frame your words in a constructive way. Female athletes want to hear a full explanation of what they are being asked to do; they want to understand their coaches' expectations. As the Woman's Sports Foundation reports, "The female athletes we spoke to wanted to feel like they could talk to their coach about anything. They acknowledged that they often wanted to know 'why' more than male athletes and demanded more discussion." Your female athletes want you to talk to them, and they will listen to what you have to say, as long as you say it in a way that doesn't make them feel defensive or small.

Louisa, a young basketball player I worked with, complained to me that her private school coach would never give her team a full explanation of new techniques they were learning. When she tried to take him aside to ask him questions, he just brushed her off. Her frustration was evident as she struggled with this situation. Eventually, she was industrious enough to ask other players and coaches for help, and eventually she obtained the information she was looking for. But not all young women are as resilient as Louisa; faced with the same situation, many young players might simply give up and quit the team.

As I've said already, providing positive, constructive feedback is not the same as coddling your athletes. Knowing what we know about female psychology, it's clear that girls and women don't respond well to being berated. So why not lift your players up by giving positive praise when it's deserved rather than dragging them down by nitpicking every mistake? Why not tell your players what problems you're seeing and make suggestions for how they can change their behaviors without using super-harsh and reactive words, if that's more effective than yelling? If the goal is to elicit the best possible performance from your players, keeping positive is really just smart strategy.

Female Athletes Tend to Underestimate and Limit Themselves

Even when getting positive feedback, girls are more likely than boys to underrate their athletic abilities. I have seen female athletes at all levels fail to realize just how talented or capable they were. Sometimes female athletes know that they are capable of more, but they intentionally or unintentionally hold themselves back. This happens because females gravitate toward being cooperative and collaborative and are very much attached to the idea of fairness. This is a wonderful quality to have in life, but in competition, fairness can be a stumbling block. Coaches should keep an eye out for girls who limit themselves because they want to be liked or don't want to hurt their peers' feelings; athletes like these need to be encouraged to push themselves and compete at the highest level they're capable of.

Female Athletes "Tend and Befriend"

C. J. Healy, an assistant basketball coach at San Rafael High School in California who coaches girls aged eight to eighteen, is another advocate of sports as a form of empowerment for girls and women. She believes that team play and hard work build self-confidence and empower girls to succeed in life. Her philosophy is to create the opportunity for girls to perform at their best. She sees sports as a metaphor for life. She wants her girls to learn life lessons and skills such as coping with loss and success, developing sportsmanship, setting goals, and finding inner strength. Her role is to guide them to trust themselves and develop self-confidence. I quietly chuckled to myself as she described how one girl's success in making a basket triggered her to burst into such tears of joy that she had to be pulled out of the game to calm down. C.J. shared, "Girls have so many emotional things to deal with."

When we spoke, Healy explained why it's so important to focus on the psychological elements of the game with girls. She helps them to learn mental toughness through dealing with disappointment on the court and strategies for moving on emotionally from the last basket or out-of-bounds ball. C.J. believes that preparation for the game is even more important than the game itself. In terms of athletic females' relationships, she recognizes girls tend to group up and hang out together, showing mutual respect and a belief in fairness, and they are emotional on and off the court.

Coach Healy learned about empowering women from her feminist mom. Her Canadian family lived in Nova Scotia and encouraged her and her three athletic sisters to participate in sport. Her youngest sisters, who were twins, were both on the national sailing team, with one even being on the Olympic sailing team. In her collegiate years, she played basketball, and her middle sister rowed. All the sisters supported each other. While working on her master's degree, she participated in a project called "Futures for Women in Sport," which aimed primarily to promote the empowerment of girls through athletics. Clearly, then, Healy learned early on that cooperation and collaboration among women is essential, and now she's passing that knowledge on through her coaching. Coaching her eight-year-old daughter's basketball team is a delight for her. She enjoys watching the girls she coaches grow and expand through the teamwork of basketball.

In your coaching, keep in mind the tend-and-befriend model of female reactions to stress. Girls may not respond well to heavy confrontation when conflicts arise. They prefer to sit down and talk (tend and befriend) when something stressful or upsetting occurs rather than to engage in direct confrontation (the fight-or-flight approach). In *Catch Them Being Good*, Tony DiCicco describes one incident in which Mia Hamm told him to leave another player alone during a game. He felt she was showing a "lack of respect," so he yelled back a few unpleasant words and got on her case soon afterward when she made a mistake. Visibly distressed by the exchange, she carried her upset into halftime. DiCicco was inclined to pull her from the game, but at team captain Carla Overbeck's suggestion, he kept her in. Later, DiCicco met with Hamm, admitted that he had been overcoaching, and apologized; Hamm apologized back, and the dispute was laid to rest. In other words, DiCicco approached his players with a tend-and-befriend mind-set, and because of that they were able to move past an issue that might otherwise have festered and grown.

Every single coach who works with female athletes needs to keep the issues we've just gone over in mind. Certain biological imperatives directly influence girls' and women's behaviors in sport: a need for emotional connections, a preference for cooperating and collaborating with and pleasing others, a proclivity toward empathy, intuitiveness, a penchant for positive peer-group camaraderie, and a desire to have fun. A coach's job is to bring out the best in every player by taking these qualities into account.

EMPOWERING FEMALE ATHLETES

Lindsay Gottlieb, who coaches the University of California, Berkeley's women's basketball team, is the model of a coach who understands what makes women tick and how to bring out their best performances. She describes her coaching style as "authentic" and "educational," and says she believes in setting up a foundation of trust as the first step toward building a great team. "The most effective way to coach is to start and end games with a positive attitude," she says. She focuses on being reasonable, calm, measured, and trusting with her players and on cultivating a "team-first" mentality: she lets her players know that the decisions made on the court are always about the team as a whole performing its best, not about personal successes.

As much as she values teamwork, however, Lindsay also values individual empowerment. She works on building leadership qualities in her players. In 2013, in addition to having the usual three senior captains, she also made a junior, Reshanda Gray, a captain in an effort to reach out to the younger girls on the team. Reshanda's aptitude for leadership shows in her enthusiastic and affectionate coaching style. She made it out of South Central Los Angeles, one of the toughest parts of the city, with her signature smile intact, and she's kept that positivity going through the years. Lindsay also teaches her young women how to handle themselves off the court—with media and staff, for example—and encourages them to have fun. In April 2013, following that year's seasonal Final Four participation, the team made a music video that they wrote, produced, and starred in, titled "Started from the Bottom (Now We're Here)." As for Lindsay herself, what matters most to her and her staff, she says, is that their players "know that we care about them as people and help them to perform their best."

THE ATHLETIC TRIANGLE

In coaching teenage and youth girls, we commonly encounter what is considered the athletic triangle: the relationship between the coach, the parents, and the athletic girls. The key ingredient in making this triangle work is active and clear communication; the problem is that all three points of the triangle have to be willing to work together for this to be possible. Part of coaching girls is including moms and dads as well.

We've all heard loud, critical parents in the stands, screaming at their children about everything that they're doing wrong, and we've seen those kids cringe with shame and humiliation. These are the most difficult parents to deal with. However, with some work, they can sometimes change. I've seen it firsthand. One of my clients, a seventeen-year-old volleyball player named Gabby, told me during one session that she appreciated her dad coming to all her games, but he often yelled negative, critical things that were not helpful and embarrassed her in front of her team. We brought her dad in for a couple of sessions to discuss the situation, and it turned out he didn't even realize how upsetting (or loud) his yelling was. Once he became aware of his behavior, he started working to modify it, and eventually he calmed down enough that Gabby rarely heard his voice from the stands anymore. When that happened, her level of play improved significantly.

The first step in dealing with problem situations involving a coach, a parent, or an athlete is recognizing that the athletic triangle exists. According to the Women's Sports Foundation, there are two types of athletic triangles: the professional and the developmental. In the professional model, only the parents' and coach's wishes are considered, and the young female athlete's feelings and desires are disregarded altogether. In the developmental model, in contrast, the focus is on the young female athlete; the role of the coach is to give guidance, support, and instruction and to let the parents know what level of involvement they should have and what their responsibilities are. The role of the parents, meanwhile, is to provide active support.

The developmental model of the athletic triangle supports female athletes' need for connection, bonding, and collaboration. The professional model does just the opposite: denying female youth athletes a say in their training does not allow them to develop the intimate peer relationships essential to creating a cohesive team. A Greek study that explored the athletic triangle demonstrated "that effective co-ordination of parental support and a collaborative relationship with a coach provide an optimal platform for an athlete's development."[3] The study, which looked at five athletic triangles in which all the athletes were teen female swimmers, also concluded that each member of every triangle was equally aware of the interpersonal issues at play, including the need for trust and respect, a feeling of commitment, and a positive coordination of the relationship behaviors of coach, athlete, and parents. Support emerged as a primary factor.

Articles that caution parents about letting their girls participate in sports at all pop up frequently, but much of this material is unnecessary fearmongering. The benefits of sports participation far outweigh the detriments; as you will hear from most coaches, playing sports builds character, teaches discipline, provides structure, and gives girls something fun to be a part of. Playing sports only becomes a negative experience when parents or coaches deviate from the developmental model of the athletic triangle.

A parent's responsibilities when it comes to supporting their young female athlete include the following:

- Recognizing her right and desire to participate in sports
- Respecting her and her decision to play sports
- Listening to her and validating her feelings
- Keeping track of her participation and attending her games, meets, or events
- Communicating periodically with her coach
- Trusting her coach and refraining from being too intrusive
- Admitting to mistakes
- Accepting and embracing her performance, no matter what
- Supporting and hearing her when she doesn't perform as well as she wanted to

- Being a model of sportsmanship so that she has a positive role model for her own behavior[4]

When coaches, parents, and athletes work to get along, like, and respect each other, we are likely to see more cooperation and better performances follow close behind. One parent frequently comments, "I really enjoyed watching you play," which expresses support no matter what the outcome. Numerous studies validate taking this positive but neutral attitude.

In more complicated situations, there are times when a sports psychologist can work as an additional resource, though weaving a fourth member into the triangle is always tricky (a triangle has only three points, after all!). However, it is sometimes necessary to get an outsider's input. A sports psychologist has significant training and experience in working with athletes and athletic teams, holding a PhD in either sports sciences or sports/clinical psychology, a state license, and certification through the Association of Applied Sports Psychology (AASP). These professionals are trained to deal with everything from family intervention and performance enhancement to injuries to more serious psychological problems such as anxiety and depression. The sports psychologist may or may not communicate directly with the coach(es), depending on the situation, but he or she will always communicate directly with the parents.

COACHING GIRLS VERSUS BOYS

There's no getting around it: females and males are different, both psychologically and biologically. Mike Woitalia, a sports journalist and youth coach, has both written about soccer and coached under-thirteen girls. He's observed the girls wanting to group up on the same team, continually talk, and socialize. By allowing them to enjoy themselves, he hopes to create a passion for soccer. He, like all the coaches in this chapter, takes the best approach when working with girls—a positive one. Girls and women experience relationships as intimate and emotional, and their primary interest is in connecting, collaboration, self-management, intuition, empathy, concern for others, fairness, and having fun. This means that in order for an athletic triangle involving a female athlete to be successful, both parents and coaches must honor these unique needs.

That's why coaches who keep female athletes' mental processes and preferences in mind are so much more successful than those who don't. Ultimately, acknowledging and accepting these differences and implementing a positive approach is a win for both coaches and the female athletes they work with.

TEN MENTAL STRATEGIES FOR COACHING FEMALE ATHLETES

1. Remember that female athletes view relationships from an emotional viewpoint both culturally and biologically.
2. Build a positive relationship with female athletes by talking and listening to them.
3. Remember that girls and women do their best work in a circle, not in a top-down hierarchy.
4. Learn to push female athletes hard without resorting to yelling negative comments.
5. Remember that female athletes often "tend and befriend" when overstressed and avoid heated confrontations when issues arise.
6. Develop trust and positive motivation and build your players' self-confidence.
7. Encourage friendships between teammates on and off the court to create a more positive, cohesive team on the court.
8. Help female athletes learn to value themselves through their sport.
9. Teach female athletes that cooperation, collaboration, and competition can all work together.
10. Find ways to have fun, even with higher-level female athletes.

9

PIONEERING FEMALE ATHLETES LAID THE FOUNDATION

When women bond together, they become powerful enough to move mountains. This is evident when we reflect back on pioneering women athletes. Looking at the conditions women competed under during the 1960s and those they compete under today, it's clear that the changes early female athletes made within the world of sports were both enormous and enduring. Thanks to these pioneering women, the 2012 US Olympic team had 267 women—6 more than the team's 261 men—and although men outnumbered women at the 2014 Sochi games, there were still 105 women on the US team (only a handful fewer than the 118 men). In skeleton competition at Sochi, we even watched a thirty-one-year-old mother of two win a silver medal—additional evidence of the progress we've made over the past fifty years.

Coinciding with the feminist movement of the 1960s, famous female athletes banded together to work toward establishing equal rights for pro women in sports. Just before the passage of Title IX in 1972, a courageous group of professional female tennis players, led by Billie Jean King and Rosie "Rosebud" Casals, took a stand against the US Tennis Association (USTA) about the pay discrepancy between female and male tennis players. This group of women, called the "Original Nine," decided to take the USTA on, and the result was the creation of the Virginia Slims Tour and eventually the Women's Tennis Association, which celebrated its fortieth birthday in 2012. Today, professional female and male tennis players get equal pay, all because of that group of committed, connected women players who demanded fair treatment for themselves and their fellow female athletes. Together, the Original Nine proved that when women connect and rally together, they empower each other and operate at their strongest.

PRE–TITLE IX ATHLETE PIONEERS

Before Billie Jean King and her peers began to advocate for female athletes, the sports world had a far different landscape. In 1964, for example, Olympic swimmer Donna de Varona found herself out in the cold when it came to college scholarships, despite the fact that she had just set world records and received two gold medals at that year's Olympic Games. Through her persistence, she did manage to land a job as a sportscaster for ABC's *Wild World of Sports* in the 1960s at the tender age of seventeen and became an advocate for and avid supporter of Title IX. Six years later, even after passage of the legislation, "an estimated 50,000 men were attending US colleges and universities on athletic scholarships," while "fewer than 50 women" could claim the same privilege. [1]

Many young women today don't understand what an enormous impact Title IX has had on their sporting lives, but the truth is that prior to its passage, female athletes had few rights or opportunities. There were no athletic scholarships, they earned far less as professionals than male athletes, and women were discouraged from playing certain sports; essentially, women were still being treated as second-class citizens, both inside and outside of the world of sports. While in high school in 1973, Ann Meyers Drysdale's talents as a basketball player were recognized, and she became the first young woman to receive a full four-year scholarship at a Division I school, the University of California, Los Angeles.

When I was in high school in the late 1960s and early 1970s, some sports were regarded as "too masculine," and girls who played them were automatically labeled as lesbians. At my high school, field hockey players and my Girl Scout backpacking group fell into that category; meanwhile, the Girl's League (which did stuff "tomboys" regarded as "girly") was considered cool. I was the vice president of the Girls' League and helped put on an annual fashion show. At the time, the only sports deemed "ladylike" were horseback riding, figure skating, tennis, and badminton. A competitive swimmer like Donna de Varona was a fish out of water in the 1960s. No wonder she was treated like such a special case; no wonder she wasn't offered any scholarships despite her impressive Olympic performance. No one knew what to do with her.

Even so, a number of pioneers came before de Varona, including Babe Didrikson (Olympian in track and field in the 1930s and professional golfer in the 1940s and 1950s) and Wilma Rudolph (three-time Olympic gold medalist in track and field in 1960). A behind-the-scenes women's sports advocate was Dr. Carole Oglesby (PhD in kinesiology and PhD in counseling). Carole grew up in a sports-focused family: her dad played semipro baseball and was an avid golfer, and her mother was an enthusiastic high school basketball player. Carole's passion for sport showed up in her lifelong commitment to it. Oglesby, a highly motivated, ambitious, and high-energy team builder, played on an all-girls softball team in the 1950s. Collaboration and bonding were always important to her; she valued the closeness she shared with her team members, and in fact she is still friends with teammates from that team at age seventy-six. She was also very competitive (she describes herself as always having experienced a lot of "competitive anxiety"). As a visionary, she views the roles of collaboration and bonding as essential to female athletes.

Oglesby attended UCLA from 1957 to 1964, receiving both her bachelor's and master's there before going on to Purdue for a PhD. Her dissertation focused on the social-cultural dimensions of sport; she also spent a third of her time there teaching women's/gender studies. When she began working in sports psychology in the 1970s, the field was dominated by men, but she persisted, and in 1981 she received a full professorship to Temple University. Since then, she has dedicated her life to national and global women's sport advocacy, especially improving the position of collegiate women in athletics. She has always displayed a friendly, curious, empathic, intuitive, and forward-thinking attitude about women in sport, and she recognizes and supports female athletes need to bond and collaborate with each other. Through these relationships, she says, female athlete's can empower themselves and others and succeed in sports and life. In 1989, Carole embarked on a ten-year journey: she began working on her PhD in counseling. Working full-time as a tenured professor, she diligently progressed through this program, finishing in 1999. Persistence and tenacity are two of her remarkable qualities.

She has dedicated the last twenty years of her life to national and global women's sport advocacy. Relationships are highly important to her. She has appreciated her closest confidants' support for her visions and help in realizing them. She has spent her entire career working toward the improved position of collegiate women in sport. She encourages female athletes to empower and succeed in sports and life.

Carole was one of my role models. We met through AASP in the early 1990s. The truly remarkable part of Carole's personality was her constant friendliness and encouragement to stay with sports psychology despite the many years it has taken me to mature and develop as a sports psychologist. At each convention I attended, her manner remained the same, always friendly and welcoming. Carole has remained a role model for many women over the years. She fights for what she believes in and still retains her down-to-earth manner. Seeing Carole annually at AASP was one of the reasons that I kept going back.

Support continues to be an important vehicle for female athletes. Many pioneers didn't necessarily recognize it, as such, but they clearly experienced it. Without these pioneers and their efforts to move women athletes' rights along, we wouldn't be increasing our numbers in sport. According to both the 2013 National Sporting Goods Association Participation Study and the American Bicyclist Study, "1.2 million fewer males participated in bicycle riding while 1.3 million more females did ride a bicycle in 2012 compared to 2011."[2] Each year, more females enter the sports world. By learning about pioneering women and the establishment of women's sports groups, we can observe how much our emotional relationships, psychological tendencies, and brains influence us in our athletic pursuits. We need to understand some of the history that has allowed us to participate in sports. Now, we can fully see the road ahead in our need to be recognized for our unique strengths in emotionally based relationships and the mind and brain workings that go along with our sports participation.[3]

PRE–TITLE IX ATHLETES BOND TOGETHER

Prior to Title IX, female athletes had few rights. There were no athletic scholarships, male and female pro athletes did not enjoy equity in pay, and women were still treated as second-class citizens in the world of sports. In fact, they were not even allowed to participate in certain types of sporting events due to the false belief that they were physically fragile.

Kathrine Switzer is another female athlete who pursued her athletic dreams at a time when it was difficult for women to do so. In 1967, despite the fact that women were not technically allowed to enter the race, twenty-year-old Switzer ran the Boston Marathon. She registered as K. V. Switzer, a twenty-year-old Syracuse University student. When Jock Semple, one of the race's organizers, saw that Switzer was a woman, he jumped off the media truck and attempted to physically remove her from the marathon. Arnie Briggs, Switzer's coach, tried and failed to pull Semple off her. Seeing that Briggs was having trouble, Switzer's 235-pound boyfriend, Tom Miller, threw a cross body block that sent Semple flying. Semple's attack scared Kathrine half to death, but his actions made her more determined than ever: "I'm going to finish this race on my hands and knees if I need to," she told the men supporting her. Ultimately, she finished the race in four hours, twenty minutes. Still, women were not allowed to officially register for and run the race until 1972—five years later.

TENNIS ATHLETES TAKE A STAND

During this same time, the Original Nine decided to band together and challenge the US Tennis Association about the widening gap between women's and men's treatment in sports. Most tournaments at the time paid women eight to ten times less than men, and many female pros wanted better facilities, prize money, general support, and media coverage for their sports. They were angered by the argument that male players should earn more as they were "the breadwinners" for their families. Some pro female tennis players, like Billie Jean King and her doubles partner, Rosie Casals, wanted to challenge the USTA and create a series of tournaments specifically for women; others, like Margaret Court, Evonne Goolagong, and Chris Evert, were hesitant to take such a radical stand.

Finally, King and Casals took the bull by the horns: they recruited seven other female pro tennis players—Julie Heldman (daughter of Gladys), Nancy Richey, Kerry Melville, Peaches Bartkowicz, Kristy Pigeon, Judy Dalton, and Valerie Ziegenfuss—to band together with them, and King used her influence to reach out and get the attention of Gladys Heldman, editor of *World Tennis Magazine*, the major tennis publication at that time. In 1970, all nine women signed $1 contracts with *World Tennis Magazine*. Heldman reached out to her friend Joe Cullman, CEO of Philip Morris, and he agreed to sponsor the first all-women's tennis tour. With the slogan "You've come a long way, baby," the Virginia Slims Tour (which offered much better prize money and conditions than the USTA's tournaments) was born, and King and her eight fellow revolutionaries were thrilled. This wasn't just about money; it was also about the empowerment and rights of women as a group. Our empathic, intuitive, and collaborative nature was put to the challenge. This group of brave and committed women led the way for girls and women in sport to start demanding equal treatment.

At the same time as the Original Nine were fighting for women's rights in tennis, Representative Patsy T. Mink (Hawaii), Representative Edith Green (Oregon), Senator Birch Bayh (Indiana), Dr. Bernice Sandler, and Donna Lopiano, former CEO of the Women's Sports Foundation (WSF) were all actively working for the passage of Title IX. The legislation was originally intended to support women's rights in education overall, not just in athletics. Little did the originators realize one of the greatest areas of impact would be high school and collegiate women's sports. The original legislation, in fact, made little mention of sports whatsoever.

Despite the fact that Title IX did not have direct ties to girls' participation in sports, a handful of famous athletes, including Billie Jean King and Donna de Varona, advocated for it. Donna de Varona talked about her role in supporting the legislation: "I was part of a family of women that have made a difference that started in the sixties and seventies competing at times when women's rights were hard fought. Sports was about the socialization process and the values you learn on the field of play."

Title IX's basic premise was as follows: "No person in the United States shall, on the basis of sex, be excluded from participation in, be denied the benefits of, or be subjected to discrimination under any educational program or activity receiving Federal financial assistance." King and de Varona recognized the potential there. Together with other prominent women athletes who supported Title IX, they did much to help ensure its passage.

IN THE WAKE OF TITLE IX: ANN MEYERS DRYSDALE

Despite initial resistance to Title IX and its slow implementation, some young women benefited from the new law almost immediately. Ann Meyers Drysdale was an up-and-coming basketball player when Title IX was passed. In 1974, she became the first high school player to make the US national team; in 1975, she played on the gold-medal-winning Pan American team; and in 1976 she played for the first Olympic women's basketball team, which took home a silver medal that year. Remarkably, she signed on as a free agent with the Indiana Pacers, a National Basketball Association team, in 1979, though she wasn't selected for the final team. Eventually, Meyers Drysdale, once a shy and unassuming young woman, entered the world of broadcasting: she called the 1984 Olympics for ABC.

Asked about her mentors and role models, Meyers Drysdale described a long list of significant people who influenced and helped her as an athlete and a leader, including tennis pioneer Billie Jean King, Olympic double-gold-medaling track-and-field runner Wilma Rudolph, and Babe Didrikson, a 1932 Olympic gold and silver medalist, basketball player, and professional golfer. In terms of coaching, Ann named her coach during her senior year at UCLA, Billie Moore; Sue Gunter, assistant coach of the 1976 Olympic basketball team; and, of course, UCLA's legendary and iconic coach, whom she called PaPa, John Wooden. One of Ann's favorite quotes is from Wooden: "Failing to prepare is preparing to fail."

Meyers Drysdale's philosophy about relationships in sports is that it's always important to help and support your teammates. Doing so, she says, takes courage and hard work. Ann's viewpoint echoes Winston Churchill's: "Failure is not fatal, success is not final, it's the courage that counts."

POST–TITLE IX BREAKTHROUGHS

In the 1970s and 1980s, following passage of Title IX, a number of organizations geared toward supporting girls' and women's involvement in sports sprang up. Two of these, the Women's Sports Foundation and the Women's Mountain Bike and Tea Society (WOMBATS), particularly embody the values most integral to female athletes' success.

The Women's Sports Foundation

Though Donna de Varona did not win any scholarships after her incredible performance at the 1964 Olympics, she did manage to land a job as a sportscaster for ABC's *Wild World of Sports* soon afterward. Through that position she met Billie Jean King, and the two athletes became friends. With de Varona's, Casals's, and many others' help and input, King founded the Women's Sports Foundation in San Francisco in 1974 to support girls and young women in growing and developing their lives through participation in sports. The WSF has been teaching leadership skills, protecting Title IX rights, and shining a spotlight on women's sports ever since.[4]

To start up the WSF, King lent her well-known name to the organization to establish credibility and donated $5,000 of her own money. De Varona, meanwhile, used her numerous contacts in broadcasting to reach out for assistance. The WSF's first office space, in San Mateo, California, was donated. The first advisory board, which consisted primarily of famous Olympic and pro female athletes—Jane Blalock (pro golfer), Donna de Varona (Olympic gold medalist swimmer), Chris Evert (number one pro tennis player), Diane Holum (Olympic gold medalist speed skater), Joan Joyce (softball player, pro golfer, national basketball team player, and coach), Micki King (Olympic gold medalist diver), Karen Logan (Women's Basketball Association player), Sandy Poulsen (Olympic alpine skier), Paula Sperber (pro bowler), and Wyomia Tyus (Olympic gold medalist in track and field)—was established a couple of years later. Ann Meyers Drysdale also threw her support behind the WSF, citing the invaluable role that guidance from others played in her own life as her inspiration to get involved.

Whether or not they realized that their efforts were emblematic of women's affiliative nature, these pioneering female athletes merged together in a "circle" and did what they felt most comfortable doing: they talked to one another, listened to each other's viewpoints, and created something great through collaboration. Since its inception, the Women's Sports Foundation has created numerous life-changing programs and has become a significant presence in the promotion and support of girls and women in sports.

The WOMBATS

Jacquie Phelan, often referred to as the "godmother of women's mountain biking," founded the Women's Mountain Bike and Tea Society in Marin County, California, in 1987 to encourage girls' and women's participation in the sport, which until then had been dominated by men. The WOMBATS consists of a network of women, aged twenty-one or older, who share a passion for pedaling in the dirt.

Like so many female athletes of the 1980s, Phelan rode and raced in primarily a "man's" sport. She described her role perfectly, saying that she had become "a sort of honorary man, or had my own in-between gender, since 'no woman could ride like that' (amazing to hear that kind of sentence thirty years later, but there are still plenty of concrete ceilings around keeping the ladies down)."

In 1985 Phelan became the first US mountain bike racer (male or female) to compete abroad, when she traveled to Wales to participate in a crazy event called the Man versus Horse Marathon, which primarily included runners and horses. The race began in 1980 as the result of a bet between two men in a pub in the small town of Llanwrtyd Wells. The two men began arguing about whether a man was capable of outrunning a horse in a long-distance race. The owner of the pub, Gordon Green, decided that the argument needed testing in public, and the Man versus Horse Marathon was born. The race is run over rough terrain, including up and down hills, through fields, across streams, and, of course, through the bogs. For a few years, the event included mountain bikes, and Phelan, a champion women's cyclist in the United States at the time, traveled to this little burg for the fun and challenging event. She narrowly lost to the first horse but did manage to win the "human" part of the race.

Phelan had got the idea for the WOMBATS after riding with a group of fourteen women on Mother's Day in 1984. She thought it would be a great idea for women to ride together and not worry about all the "macho stuff" they had to deal with when they rode with men.[5] Two years after the Wales marathon, she decided to realize her dream of a women-only mountain biking group. She decided that she would "serve up a dish of fat tire fun to women." Phelan established the WOMBATS so that more women could experience and learn the sport of mountain biking. The group places emphasis on the importance of riders "staying in touch with their excellent intuitive voice," having patience with themselves, meeting other women riding partners, and, importantly, not being put down for riding slow or not keeping up. Through the WOMBATS, Phelan created a place for women of all levels of mountain biking skills to meet up, share a social experience, and learn more about the sport. WOMBATS directed female athletes' energy toward the collaborative and communicative nature of women during a time when awareness about the importance of these traits was limited. Today, the group has expanded greatly and has branches in many other states.

PIONEERING ATHLETES IN THE POST–TITLE IX YEARS

Women's sports began to grow in popularity in the 1980s. In both track and field and soccer, American female athletes came charging through the gate. Jackie Joyner-Kersee, a heptathlete and long jumper, took the 1987 World Championships and 1988 Olympics by storm. She walked away with two gold medals in both events. *Sports Illustrated* eventually dubbed her the "Greatest Female Athlete of the 20th Century." Her sister-in-law, Florence Griffith Joyner (nicknamed Flo Jo), a three-time gold medalist in the 1988 Seoul Olympic Games, is still considered by many the fastest woman of all time as she still holds the world records in the one hundred and two hundred meters. These women stood out as role models for the younger generation—as female athletes young girls could look up to, admire, and use as inspiration.

During the 1980s, soccer was at the top of the list as well. The sport got help from Title IX and from the creation of the first national women's team in 1985. In 1987, the "Fab Five"—Julie Foudy, Brandi Chastain, Joy Biefeld (Fawcett), Kristine Lilly, and Mia Hamm (who was only fifteen at the time)—led the way in joining the national team. In 1991, the team won the first Women's World Cup. In the ensuing years, these women bonded, collaborated, communicated effectively, used their intuitive nature, and supported each other with a commitment that provides a role model for all young female athletes today, no matter what their sport. In 1999, after the national team became gold medalists in the World Cup, Kristine Lilly and the team realized that something big had happened on and off the field for girls in sports. "After a while," Mia Hamm said in 2004, "it wasn't about soccer anymore. It's what brought us together; it's not what will keep us together." They went on to win gold in the 2004 Athens Olympic Games before Hamm, Foudy, Fawcett, and Chastain eventually retired in 2005.

Kristine Lilly was the longest-playing member of the Fab Five, with twenty-three years on the national team (1987–2010). After taking time off in 2008 to have her first daughter, Sidney, Lilly came back only five months after giving birth to play in the final two games of the season. Her accomplishments in her twenty-four-year career include 352 international appearances, active play in four different decades, and being both the youngest and the oldest player on the US soccer team to score a goal. In 2011, she retired and gave birth to her second daughter, Jordan, on September 2 of that year.

In a recent interview, Kristine depicted herself as intrinsically motivated, hardworking, consistent, and caring about others, especially her teammates. She said her athletic family, particularly her brother, inspired, encouraged, and pushed her to participate and improve in sports. She remembers the early years of playing on the national team as a bunch of young kids having a good time and says the friendships she forged with Julie Foudy, Mia Hamm, Joy Fawcett, and Brandi Chastain have been long lasting. She still feels that she could turn to any of them for support and help, just as she did during their soccer-playing years.

Today, Lilly works to instill self-confidence in the young athletes she coaches at her camps. She says it's important to keep in mind that girls want to please their coaches and know that you care about them; they want do well and be singled out for praise or criticism privately; and they experience embarrassment more easily than boys. Asked to rank the top three people who influenced her in soccer, Anson Dorrance, the coach who first invited her to join the national team, immediately emerged as number one. The other two influences she cited were groups: her Fab Five teammates and her family. Kristine's affinity for her family and old friends speaks volumes about the emotionality with which females approach relationships. As Kristine states on her website, "A fun and creative environment will bring out the best in everyone!"

Diana Nyad, a pioneering long-distance swimmer, has relied on her own support network throughout her life to accomplish incredible feats in her career as well. For ten years, from 1969 to 1979, Nyad was the greatest endurance swimmer in the world. In 1975, she earned the world speed record when she swam around Manhattan (twenty-eight miles) in a record-breaking seven hours, fifty-seven minutes. In 1978, at twenty-nine years old, she attempted to swim from Cuba to Florida but was unable to finish due to poor weather conditions. Just a year later, in 1979, she swam from North Bimini, Bahamas, to Juno Beach, Florida. Nyad completed the 102-mile course in an amazing twenty-seven hours, thirty minutes, averaging a strong 3.7 miles per hour and setting a world record for both women and men in open-water swimming. In each of these swims, a crew on a boat accompanied her the whole way.

The support of her relationships was essential to these earlier successes. After her Bahamas-Florida swim, she retired and pursued a career in broadcasting and journalism. She chose the role of women's rights advocate and continued supporting women in sports as she involved herself with the Women's Sports Foundation. She served as a WSF trustee for years and remains involved as one of the foundation's "athletes" today.

In 2007, after her mother died, Diana took a good long look at her life and decided to try the Cuba-Florida swim once again. She has given us a model for how belief in oneself can make all the difference. She was no longer as physically fast as she had been in her twenties, but she believed that her mind was much stronger, especially in terms of her powers of concentration and perspective on life. Despite three failed attempts between 2010 and 2011, she persisted and never gave up on achieving her "extreme dream." On September 2, 2013, on her fifth attempt (at age sixty-four), she became the first person to swim nonstop (and without a shark cage) from Cuba to Florida. It took her fifty-two hours, fifty-three minutes to complete the swim.

Good conditions and her strong mind were instrumental in this achievement (her mantra leading up to the record-breaking swim was "Find a way!"). She had many tricks up her sleeve: for instance, she carried eighty-five songs in her head, which she silently sang to herself as she swam. She also gives much of the credit for her success to her crew, which accompanied her on a boat during the swim (she was accompanied by such a crew during every long-distance swim she ever did). In interviews following her Cuba-Florida swim, Nyad showed great respect and gratitude toward her crew, acknowledging their efforts to help make her dream come true over and over again. Her best friend of thirty years and business partner, Bonnie Stoll, also supported Diana the whole way through all of her attempts.

Diana's inspiring accomplishment is a shining example of the importance of never giving up, using all of your power, and persisting until you succeed. She provides a model for older women in sports in particular. We can learn much from her, especially to persevere, aim to finish, and not hesitate to assemble a team for support, which we women athletes need. A big part of our achievements involves the supporting cast around us.

Diana's advice to others included three important messages:

1. You should never, ever give up.
2. You are never too old to chase your dreams.
3. Even when it looks like a solitary sport, it's a team effort.

Since 1973, we've gone from only thirty thousand high school female athletes in the whole United States to well over three million. Young women's participation in collegiate sports has increased sixfold, and today thousands of scholarships are granted to female athletes each year, a huge improvement over the mere fifty granted in 1973. According to Dr. Oglesby, who is now considered the grandmother of sports psychology, much of this is due to women's sports organizations, which she says have become "an empowerment vehicle for women in sports." And it makes sense that women would achieve so much through collaboration: women not only find comfort in groups, but seem to be more energized to stand up to challenges when surrounded by peers, just as Shelley Taylor's "tend-and-befriend" model asserts. It should come as no surprise that the great strides female athletes have made in the past forty years have been the result of their coming together and working side by side. Diana Nyad's personal and project-oriented supporters supported her from pre-swim until she walked onto the beach in Key West. Her team helped her prove that you're never too old to achieve your dreams (even athletic ones). The power of the human spirit should never be underestimated.

The role of collaboration and verbal communication for women is important to understand because these were critical to opening sports up to female athletes. The female athletes discussed in this chapter all have in common their shared emphasis on teamwork and friendship. Upon completing her world-record-breaking swim in 2013, Diana Nyad immediately exclaimed, "We did it!" Kristine Lilly credits her fellow Fab Fivers with being among her biggest influences and greatest supporters. Donna de Varona has emphatically stated, "Relationships are everything!" Sixty years after playing with them, Dr. Carole Oglesby is still friends with the girls from her high school softball team. Each of these pioneering athletes clearly illustrates the importance of emotional relationships for women and provides role models for the youth of today.

In learning about pioneering women and the establishment of women's sports groups, we are able to observe how much our emotional relationships, psychological tendencies, and brains influence us in our athletic pursuits. Now that we understand the history of the individuals and organizations that have made it possible for girls and women to participate in sports, it's possible to see more fully the road still ahead of us. Female athletes have worked to broaden the participation of females in sports, both nationally and internationally, by joining forces and expressing their collaborative nature; only by continuing to do so will we make even more progress.

The discipline, collaboration, and communication, as well as the lessons about rules and regulations, winning and losing, and playing your best, that girls learn as a result of their participation in athletics are invaluable. Sports and life are a journey—and the journey is thrilling. Thanks to pioneers like Billie Jean King, Donna de Varona, Rosie Casals, Dr. Carole Oglesby, and Ann Meyers-Drysdale, who forged the way for equal pay for professional female athletes and equal opportunity for aspiring young female athletes, more girls than ever before are embarking on that journey today.

TEN MENTAL STRATEGIES FROM FAMOUS PIONEERING FEMALE ATHLETES

1. "No matter what accomplishments you make, somebody helped you." "Believe me, the reward is not so great without the struggle."—Wilma Rudolph, Olympic runner, gold (1960) and bronze (1956) medalist
2. "Speak out. Even the biggest room needs a woman's voice."—Dr. Carole Oglesby, grandmother of sports psychology

3. "Sports is about the socialization process and the values you learn on the field of play."—Donna de Varona, Olympic gold medalist swimmer, first female ABC sportscaster, first president/chairwoman of the Women's Sports Foundation

4. "To achieve in sports you first have to have a dream, and then you must act on that dream. The best athletes are those who truly enjoy what they are doing and display a tremendous amount of work ethic. They continue to persevere in spite of setbacks and never lose sight of their ultimate goal."—Diane Holum, 1968 Olympic silver medalist and 1972 gold medalist speed skater, first female coach of the Olympic female speed skating team

5. "Life is for participating, not for spectating."—Kathrine Switzer, first woman to register and run the Boston Marathon (1968)

6. "I think self-awareness is probably the most important thing toward being a champion."—Billie Jean King, number one pro tennis player, leader of the Original Nine, founder of the Women's Sports Foundation

7. "Have a good supporting cast around you."—Rosie Casals, pro tennis player, member of the Original Nine

8. "I think it's important to show children and parents how important sports are in a child's life. . . . Sports teach so much character, teamwork, leadership, self-confidence and self-esteem."—Ann Meyers Drysdale, 1976 Olympic women's basketball silver medalist, Women's Basketball League member, and vice president of the Women's National Basketball Association's Phoenix Mercury and Phoenix Suns.

9. "I am a member of a team, and I rely on the team, I defer to it, because the team, not the individual, is the ultimate champion. . . . The backbone of success is usually found in old-fashioned, basic concepts like hard work, determination, good planning, and perseverance."—Mia Hamm, 1996 Olympic women's soccer gold medalist and 1999 World Championship soccer player

10. "The glory of sport comes from dedication, determination and desire. Achieving success and personal glory in athletics has less to do with wins and losses than it does with learning how to prepare yourself so that at the end of the day, whether on the track or in the office, you know that there was nothing more you could have done to reach your ultimate goal."—Jackie Joyner-Kersee, 1988, 1992,

and 1996 Olympic gold, silver, and bronze medalist in long jump and heptathlon, *Sports Illustrated* "Greatest Female Athlete of the 20th Century"

10

FEMALE COLLABORATIVE COMPETITION
Girls Just Wanna Have Fun

Everything we've discussed about how the female mind works thus far has pointed us toward the importance of collaborative and positive approaches with female athletes. In sports participation and competition, we see again and again that most female athletes are able and more than willing to play hard, but not if it means sacrificing enjoyment of their sport. In short: girls just wanna have fun.

Today we are more aware than ever before of the strengths and idiosyncrasies of the female brain, thanks in large part to books like *The Female Brain* (2004) and *Unleash the Power of the Female Brain* (2013). The insights we've gained into the psychological and neuropsychological features of female athletes have taught us that collaborative competition is the key to helping female athletes compete most effectively, whether they are playing as individuals or on teams.

For further evidence of the importance of collaborative competition, one need look no further than the 2014 Sochi Olympic Games. Elana Meyers and Lauryn Williams's bobsledding teamwork, which won them a silver medal, was just one example of the connection, strength, and joy we saw in the faces of many female athletes who competed. We also saw the support Noelle Pikus-Pace (one of three moms) received from her husband and two daughters throughout her entire campaign and how it helped earn her an Olympic silver medal in skeleton. The affection between the women snowboarders was evidenced by their wide smiles (especially that of the Japanese bronze medalist!) and the huge hugs they gave one another after their runs.

We didn't have more female than male US Olympians at Sochi like we did at the 2012 Summer Games, but we did still manage to have 105 women out of a total of 223 athletes representing the United States. Furthermore, when you look at the medal breakdown for 2014 female Olympians, five of the nine gold medals, four of the seven silver medals, and 50 percent of the bronze medals were received by women. Of the 105 women on Team USA, 42 won Olympic medals, including our ice hockey team. Now that's collaborative competition!

Female collaborative competition is key to girls and women doing their best in sports and life. Learning to embrace our similarities, as women, will allow us to appreciate our strengths and work together more effectively. It will allow us to compete without feeling we always need to be nice and provide us permission to push hard and perform our best. It will allow us to cultivate our natural bonding instinct.

CREATING CONNECTIONS

As we've discussed, female athletes play and compete more collaboratively and cooperatively when they feel supported and like their teammates. After all, females regard their relationships from an emotional perspective. Female teams without a certain amount of emotional connection will struggle with cohesion among the players. Whether they play individual or team sports, girls are better able to take ownership of their own and other's performances when they have a sense of team unity and identity. Younger athletes especially benefit from encouragement and support, but female athletes of every age and skill level perform at their best when they feel cared about.

Even female athletes who describe themselves as independent will, when pressed, admit that they have been influenced by any number of relationships in their athletic lives. The difference with females is that their relationships, even among celebrity athletes, contain a form of emotional connection. Female Olympic and pro athletes do not always seem to realize how much group and individual relationship dynamics affect their performances, but even these high-level athletes are deeply impacted by those around them and are more likely to excel when they feel supported and heard. Although there has been debate about the number of words used daily by women and men, there is general agreement among researchers that women talk significantly more about relationships from an intimate (emotional) perspective. The primary difference in the approach to relationships is that women athletes are emotional and talkative, whereas men are cognitive and analytical.

I worked with a young runner, Susie, who was heads above everyone else on her high school team. Because of this, she did the majority of her training alone throughout high school, and it wasn't until she went to college on a track scholarship that she got to experience the fun of sharing runs with other girls in training. When she started training side by side with other girls, Susie was astounded at the difference the companionship made in her training. She developed a couple of close friends on her team, which considerably deepened her commitment; she started to feel more fulfilled by her running and to enjoy her workouts and races more than ever before. Over the course of her first year, she consistently improved her times, and she credited those improvements largely to the support she was receiving from her coaches and teammates.

Recently, I met with a group of pitchers and catchers from San Francisco State University's women's softball team; they'd been having problems during their last couple of games, but they didn't understand exactly why. When I talked to these young women, two things quickly became evident: (1) they all seemed to like each other, and (2) despite their friendliness with one another, they lacked good connections. The pitchers were so absorbed by the stress, frustration, and negativity of their poor pitching that they were unable to encourage and cheer each other on, and the catchers were getting drawn into those feelings. In addition, the girls were focusing too much on the teams they were playing against and not enough on the quality of their own team.

After we'd been chatting for a bit, one of the pitchers spoke up about a tool that she uses: she focuses on one pitch at a time, one up to bat at a time, and one inning at a time. This is actually a tool that I use myself, and I suggested to the group that everyone take this approach into the next game and practice staying in the moment. But staying in the moment wasn't necessarily going to help them connect with one another, so I asked them if they had done anything fun with each other recently. Unsurprisingly, they hadn't; they did, however, immediately respond positively to my suggestion of going out to eat together after a game or planning some other sort of bonding activity. They were eager to create that "circle" atmosphere that women are innately drawn to; they just didn't know how to verbalize that desire until I called their attention to it. Immediately, coach Cristina Byrne responded. She later reported, "I took the girls to lunch and we went out bowling and had a great time just being together and spending time off the field."

Female athletes' desire for personal connection often leads them to act as caretakers for one another, both in sports and in life. Teammates who form close bonds look out for each other in a variety of ways. For example, as Kristine Lilly commented, soccer's Fab Five first bonded over soccer, but now they are bonding around motherhood. As Berkeley basketball player Avigiel Cohen mentioned, her teammates were like sisters; they shared personal information and emotions with one another and even celebrated their participation in the Final Four of women's collegiate basketball by creating a rap video with the whole team. The lyrics, which included the lines "Started from the bottom now we're here / Started from the bottom now my whole team . . . here," reveal what a cohesive unit they thought of the team as.[1]

Clearly, female athletes not only gravitate toward personal connections but thrive as a result of them. But if they are to build these relationships (and, by extension, improve their chances for athletic success), we have to take their psychological and biological perspectives into consideration. For instance, female athletes (like all women) have considerably higher levels of oxytocin, estrogen, and dopamine, all hormones directly related to bonding. Dr. Daniel Amen has suggested the primary strengths of the female brain are collaboration, intuition, empathy, self-control, and a little worry. Notice that collaboration is high on the list. In focusing on female athletes' innate strengths, we can both bring out the best in them and keep their love for sports alive.

A remarkable current example of female collaborative competition occurs between US twin sisters Tracy and Lanny Barnes, who had both been on the 2010 Vancouver Olympic team. Apparently, Lanny became very ill during the trials for the 2014 Sochi Games with a 104-degree temperature and didn't make the team even though she had done better in World Cup events in the biathlon in the fall prior to her illness. Tracy decided to give up her spot to Lanny. Tracy watched from the sidelines and commented about their relationship: "You know that they would do anything for you and you would definitely do anything for them. When you create a close bond with the people you care about, your friends and your family, you want to help them, you want to see them do well and achieve their dreams. . . . I'm one proud sister."[2]

BALANCING OUR SKILLS TO CREATE COLLABORATIVE COMPETITION

"Men compete and women collaborate" is an oft-used phrase, and it's true . . . but only partially. The truth is, women can both compete and collaborate, but they have to learn to balance the two. Female athletes need to learn to collaborate and compete more effectively using their abilities in language and relationships. What does this mean? Girls and women need to learn to talk and bond with each other in sports in a way that supports, encourages, and pushes them. It is possible for female athletes to push themselves to perform their best in competition while staying true to their values; they just have to find a way to talk and bond with their teammates and competitors in a way that is supportive and encouraging, yet still competitive.

The new team competition in figure skating at the Sochi Olympic Games was a good example of female skaters working for the team and themselves at the same time. If Ashley Wagner hadn't come in fourth in the short program and Gracie Gold hadn't placed second in the free skate, Team USA might not have gotten the bronze medal. In order for the team to find success, the individual members had to put forth fierce, hard-fought efforts.

In order to achieve true collaborative competition, women need to learn how to use their strengths. They must recognize that language is the tool females use to listen and absorb information. They must understand that positive relationships help cement girls and women together in sports and in life. They must ask for the verbal cues and explanations needed to improve their performances, and they must share responsibilities with teammates in order to avoid creating a pecking order. They must allow themselves to show the care, concern, and compassion they feel for other athletes (even opponents) without forgetting that they are in competition with them. They must focus positively on their skills and on building self-confidence. They must find something positive about every workout, even the bad ones.

Female athletes cannot engage in collaborative competition on their own, however; coaches need to be involved as well. Whether the team plays an individual or group sport, a solid foundation of support and connection specific to female parameters needs to be built. Talking, friendships, and the likeability of each team member are vital to young girls in sport. It's up to the leader(s), coaches, and captains to promote a feeling of inclusion within the team. Girls are tuned in to fair play and how everyone is treated, so coaches who witness interpersonal issues on the team should take the offenders aside, talk to them, and remind them that the general goal is for the group to succeed as a team. A coach needs to create an atmosphere in which every girl on the team can succeed.

THE MODEL OF FEMALE COLLABORATIVE COMPETITION

Members of a team with collaborative competition bond solidly, appreciate each other, feel listened to, commit to their sport, play their hardest, and have fun. The model of female collaborative competition consists of five key elements: talking, collaboration, cultivating positive relationships, embracing competition, and having fun. Let's explore each one.

Talking

Women and girls are highly verbal, which means that the use of language is essential for female athletes. Women like to talk to each other about their lives and are also good at listening and asking lots of questions. When we are discouraged from engaging with others in this way, we lose motivation; when allowed and encouraged to do so, in contrast, we flourish.

Women's need for spoken expression isn't limited to one aspect of sports. We see it in training and competition, on the field and off, and in many different ways. When Julia Mancuso competed in the Alpine Ladies Super Combined at Sochi and won the bronze, for example, she expressed her usual verbal exuberance and delight over winning an Olympic medal after completing her run. You don't have to watch the Olympics to witness this verbal communication; just go out to your local running trails, and you'll see women jogging along, discussing their lives (especially relationships) or perhaps strategies for the races ahead of them.

Sometimes just getting together with other female athletes, even to talk about non-sports-related issues, can be helpful for women. Look at Danelle Kabush, the pro XTERRA triathlete who set up a Facebook page so that female athletes would have a forum to discuss what it's like to be both an athlete and a mom.[3] Danelle periodically conducts interviews with young professional female XTERRA triathletes who have kids, and the athletes often mention how much it helps simply to be able to speak with other athlete moms.

If you are a female athlete, talk with your teammates or peers about your shared sport and how you got into it. Share something personal with them, and ask them questions about their own lives. When you have questions about something regarding your sport, don't hold back. Ask others to explain the details when you don't get them. Your instincts for verbal communication are a strength, not a weakness, so treat them that way; express yourself!

Collaboration

Collaboration in sports happens when two or more athletes work together to achieve a common goal. For female athletes, collaboration cements the relationships they develop with other players; it helps them bond. Sports psychologist Carole Oglesby, a strong contributor to team-building studies, describes "collaboration and bonding" as a big factor in female athletes being able to work in harmony and strive for the same goals.

Collaboration always has an emotional component for female athletes, whether they are working in a pair or on a team, with females or males. (A number of girls are introduced to sports by their brothers or fathers, and they need cooperation and collaboration with these male peers and mentors just as much as they would need them from females.) The tighter a girls' team is off the court, the better they are likely to do on the court. The US women's ice hockey team revealed what excellent collaboration they were capable of during their semifinal match against Sweden; they showed off their finesse and skill throughout the game and trounced the other team 6–1. They may not have beat Canada for the gold, but even so, we must not discount the extent to which the team worked well together throughout the rest of the tournament.

Practice bonding and collaborating with your fellow athletes, both individually and as a team. Take time to build personal relationships. Try working with other female athletes in a collaborative style. Treat this as a priority, and start right away when you join a new team or find a new training partner. Together, you can lift each other up to greater heights.

Cultivating Positive Relationships

Relationships are everything to women. Female athletes are more likely to thrive with positive relationships; we need them to achieve our personal bests in life, and that includes sports. Negative relationships make us shrink and disappear. Positive relationships, in contrast, are those in which your coaches, parents, friends, and others support you, recognize your capabilities, and provide guidance for you to achieve your goals and aspirations. Positive relationships help us grow and expand.

Athletes like Julia Mancuso exude happiness, joy, and a positive attitude. In the last three Olympics she's participated in, Julia expressed happiness over each medal that she received. She has stated, "Skiing is 99 percent mental." Remember, she had a great coach who presented her with a tiara for good luck. It's become such a part of her image that in 2010 she started an underwear line called "Kiss My Tiara," and it all began with a small gesture from a coach who was simply trying to do something positive and offer her support. In the 1999 World Championship women's soccer match, the US women won gold. Brandi Chastain fell to her knees, pulled off her shirt, and created an iconic photo that is still recognized to this day in posters across the United States. Brandi is one of the Fab Five soccer players who are all still best friends to this day. As Fab Fiver Kristine Lilly said, "I feel like I could go to any of them anytime for support if I needed it."

Two other female athletes who blossomed under the tutelage of a wonderful, positive coach are Honor Fetherston and Lisa Lopez, former competitive runners from the City College of San Francisco's cross-country team. Their coach, Ken Grace, has an upbeat, cheery, and verbally encouraging style that contributed to both women's success. He cared for Lisa and pushed her to be the best that she could be, and she went on to become the captain of Berkeley's cross-country team and an all-American miler. As for Honor, Ken's advice and positive attitude helped her to run in the Olympic trials in her forties and to become a top national Masters runner.

In the 1990s, I ran a major 50K in the pouring rain through mud. I led the race the last six miles, but it was so hard to see anything that I didn't even realize it. When I crossed the finish line, one of my training partners, Kelly (who had dropped out of the race), was waiting and cheering for me. My main goal had been to place in my age division, and I thought she was cheering as hard as she was because I had met my goal. When she told me I had won the entire race, I didn't believe it. It took her repeatedly congratulating me and telling me I had won to convince me that it was really true. I'll never forget how genuinely happy for me she was and how good it made me feel to have such heartfelt support in that moment. Throughout my ultrarunning years, Kelly and I remained friendly rivals.

I could tell you story after story about female athletes and the positive relationships around them making all the difference to their athletic success, but the message at the core of these stories is what's important: relationships are everything to females, especially female athletes. Without supportive parents, siblings, trainers, coaches, teammates, romantic partners, and friends surrounding them, female athletes simply do not have the strong foundation they need in order to become champions.

Embracing Competition

Competition is still a struggle for women. Even when we look at high-level competitors, we can see that female athletes struggle with reconciling their desire to caretake and make nice with their desire to compete and win. Girls and women who don't want to hurt others' feelings can especially be conflicted in this regard. Others may overcompensate and get too aggressive, an approach that only causes dissatisfaction and unhappiness all around. It takes work and effort, and sometimes a different perspective, to learn how to be competitive as a woman.

I myself have been guilty of letting the lessons I learned early in life about being "nice" affect the way I compete. Years ago, I was running a fifty-mile race at a pace that surprised me. As I passed the last aid station, which was 2.5 miles from the end, I looked up and spotted another woman about a mile ahead of me. I ran my guts out trying to catch up to her on a long uphill, attacking the last couple of short but steep grades at the end like mad. But just as I got close enough to really challenge the woman and possibly pass her, I backed off and didn't use my final kick. I had some fight left in me, but I didn't want to hurt her feelings by passing her just before the end of the race. I finished the race with a PR that holds to this day but ended up in eleventh place, which bummed me out at the time. I learned an important lesson from the experience: never give up pushing to perform your best.

Of course, the flip side of this is that you don't have to destroy your competition to feel that you've done your best. Wins don't just come in gold, despite what the media likes to portray. At the Sochi Olympics, the US team won so few gold medals that NBC was forced to focus on silver and bronze medalists as well (I was gratified to see more diverse coverage!). One inspiring story was that of Elana Meyers and Lauryn Williams, who made up one of the three US women's bobsled teams that competed at Sochi. Meyers and Williams were a relatively new team, but their mutual like and respect for each other were clear from the outset. Going into the final run, they were in the lead; ultimately, they lost a tiny bit of ground to the World Championship Canadian team and ended up with the silver. Rather than acting disappointed about losing the gold, however, Meyers and Williams showed great excitement at receiving a silver medal, offering up lots of smiles and positive comments in the interviews they gave afterward.

Competition is a part of being an athlete, but if you have trouble with the idea of beating other people, try to approach it as a personal challenge. Competition can be described in many different ways, after all. It's not just about winning or losing; there are many shades of gray in between. You can think of it as a way of supporting your team, developing your skills, improving yourself in some way, or playing to your potential.

Sports can teach you about setting goals and striving for more. So discover what motivates you, internally and externally. Choose the sport(s) in which you have the most skill. Face competition head-on, and be willing to take risks, knowing that only by doing so will you grow as an athlete and a person. Think of your sport as a mirror of your life, remembering that how you perform is a reflection of how you live. Practice commitment to yourself and your team, if you have one. If necessary, use a variety of tools to build up your self-confidence. Remind yourself that competition is not personal, and trying to win doesn't mean you're out to hurt others' feelings or annihilate them.

In the end, whether you are a top-level athlete competing in a tournament or a high school athlete trying for a PR, your real goal should be to push yourself as far as you can, both mentally and physically, to achieve great results. No matter what you do, not everyone is going to like you, but when you give it your all, they will at least respect you. Embrace competition as if it's an important part of you—because it is.

Having Fun

The song "Girls Just Wanna Have Fun" aptly sums up the final piece of the model of female collaborative competition. Elana Meyers was having fun as she laughed and goofed around after receiving the silver medal, and other female athletes should take their cue from her: we need to have fun in our sports at all levels of competition.

Focusing on fun is especially important for young female athletes, because it's an essential component in getting girls into sports (and keeping them interested). Just look at San Francisco State University's women's softball team, discussed earlier in this chapter. After I met with the players and encouraged them to get together to do something away from the field, coach Cristina Byrne took the young women out for a team activity. "I took the girls to lunch and we went out bowling and had a great time just being together and spending time off the field," she reported the next week. After that, she said, they started connecting with one another and got back on track.

A senior high school softball player I worked with to stop her emotional outbursts on the mound when her coach yelled negative comments about her pitching learned to disengage from his comments and continue to be positive about her game. When other teammates were up to bat, Dani and her best friend would cheer, and when others were pitching she would cheer. In shifting her attitude from a negative to a positive perspective, she had fun along with her best friend on the team.

Allowing teenage girls to focus on socializing and having fun is essential. Claudia Bouvier, a pro big-mountain and park skier (and Julia Mancuso's cousin) told me that when she was younger, her favorite coach, Ethan, was a vivacious and positive spirit who talked with her a lot. His verbal and upbeat style made it fun for her, and now she's gotten top podiums in free-skiing, slope-style, quarter-pipe, and half-pipe competitions around the world. Clearly, Ethan was doing something right.

Speak with almost any female Olympic or professional athlete, and she'll tell you stories of the fun she had with sports when she was growing up. Female athletes love to joke and laugh and have a good time with one another, and encouraging that kind of interaction can often be the key to keeping them interested and successful in their sport of choice. Victoria Yoham, a former Whole Athlete mountain bike team member, said it best: "As long as I love what I'm doing and am having fun, I'm doing my best."

CREATIVE COLLABORATION, PAST AND PRESENT

We've seen female collaborative competition for years, though we haven't always had a name for it. We've seen it in the faces of the girls who played their hearts out so their basketball team could win its only game of the year by thirty-five points; in the female tennis players who held themselves back so they could integrate another team into their structure and lift everyone up together; in the courage of the Original Nine who stood up to the US Tennis Association for more equal rights for pro women tennis players; in the commitment of the players in the first professional women's basketball league in the late 1970s; and in the deep, long-lasting friendships forged on the first US national women's soccer team.

While the general concept of female collaborative competition isn't a new one, only recently have we given it a label and begun to pinpoint its specific components. As we've done so, we've begun to acknowledge that many of women's unique traits are not weaknesses but strengths. We are not the "weaker" sex; rather, we are a different sex, one that happens to thrive on approaches that differ from those that work for male athletes. Serious female athletes train just as hard and compete with the same commitment as men, and like men, we are capable of truly great athletic feats. Unfortunately, women are still not given the same recognition or status as men, but we have made great strides since the passage of Title IX in 1972.

For female athletes in the United States, Title IX was the turning point for equal time in sports and work, and since its passage it has provided a structure and precedent for high school girls' and collegiate young women's sports to expand. Today, more and more female athletes are emerging in a wide variety of countries, even in the Middle East, where traditionally females are not allowed to show any part of their bodies in public. Globally, then, our progress has been enormous. Gone are the days when most women were forbidden from competing in certain sports because it was too "unladylike" or because we were too "fragile." Through the application of the elements of collaborative competition, we are connecting with one another and gaining ground in the sports world.

The model of female collaborative competition shows us how learning to embrace our similarities as women paves the way for appreciating and exploiting our strengths. Applying the general principles of this model allows us to compete without feeling we always need to be either nice or inordinately aggressive and gives us permission to push hard and perform to the best of our abilities. Through collaborative competition, girls and women can work together more effectively—in sports and in life.

TEN MENTAL STRATEGIES FOR ACHIEVING FEMALE COLLABORATIVE COMPETITION

1. Verbally communicate in a style that you and other players understand.
2. Be willing to listen to and exchange personal and sports information with others.
3. Work with other athletes or coaches toward common goals.
4. When not in the thick of competition, work on being friendly with your competition.
5. Remember that intimate (emotional) relationships are important to you, even in sports.
6. Surround yourself with positive relationships, and remember that a positive approach begins with you.
7. Embrace competition as a challenge to yourself.
8. Face competition head-on, and be willing to take risks.
9. Participate in fun, non-sports-related activities with other athletes.
10. Enjoy your sport, and strive to succeed.

NOTES

I. SISTERHOOD IN SPORTS

1. Louann Brizendine, *The Female Brain* (New York: Broadway Books, 2006).

2. Brizendine, *The Female Brain*.

3. Daniel G. Amen, *Unleash the Power of the Female Brain: Supercharging Yours for Better Health, Energy, Mood, Focus, and Sex* (New York: Harmony, 2013).

4. Gareth Cook, "The Secret Language Code," *Scientific American*, August 16, 2011, http://www.scientificamerican.com/article/the-secret-language-code.

5. Judith V. Jordan et al., *Women's Growth in Connection: Writings from the Stone Center* (Boston: Guilford Press, 1991).

6. Kimmel, M. "Men's Lives," *New York Times*, August 19, 2009.

7. John Cloud, "Why Girls Have BFFs and Boys Hang Out in Packs," *Time*, July 17, 2009, http://content.time.com/time/health/article/0,8599,1911103,00.html.

8. Greg Wyshynski, "Kerri Walsh Jennings and Misty May-Treanor on Their 'Marriage Counseling,'" Yahoo! Sports, July 30, 2012, https://sports.yahoo.com/blogs/fourth-place-medal/kerri-walsh-jennings-misty-may-treanor-marriage-counseling-002204382--oly.html.

9. Shelley E. Taylor et al., "Biobehavioral Responses to Stress in Females: Tend-and-Befriend, Not Fight-or-Flight," *Psychological Review* 107, no. 3 (2000): 411–29. http://taylorlab.psych.ucla.edu/2000_Biobehavioral%20responses%20to%20stress%20in%20females_tend-and-befriend.pdf.

10. Wilson Sporting Goods Co. and the Women's Sports Foundation, "The Wilson Report: Moms, Dads, Daughters and Sports," Women's Sports Foundation, June 7, 1988, https://www.womenssportsfoundation.org/en/home/research/articles-and-reports/mental-and-physical-health/moms-dads-daughters-and-sports.

11. Wilson Sporting Goods Co. and the Women's Sports Foundation, "The Wilson Report: Moms, Dads, Daughters and Sports," Women's Sports Foundation, June 7, 1988, https://www.womenssportsfoundation.org/en/home/research/articles-and-reports/mental-and-physical-health/moms-dads-daughters-and-sports.

12. Jesse A. Berlin and Susan S. Ellenberg, "Inclusion of Women in Clinical Trials," *BMC Medicine* 7 (2009), http://www.ncbi.nlm.nih.gov/pmc/articles/PMC2763864.

13. Brizendine, *The Female Brain*, 40.

14. Daniel G. Amen. *Unleash the Power of the Female Brain: Supercharging Yours for Better Health, Energy, Mood, Focus, and Sex.* (New York: Harmony, 2013).

15. "How Male and Female Brains Differ," WebMD, n.d., http://www.webmd.com/balance/features/how-male-female-brains-differ.

16. "How Male and Female Brains Differ."

2. BEST FRIENDS FOREVER

1. John Cloud, "Why Girls Have BFFs and Boys Hang Out in Packs," *Time*, July 17, 2009, http://content.time.com/time/health/article/0,8599,1911103,00.html.

2. J. E. Staurowsky et al., "Her Life Depends on It II: Sport, Physical Activity, and the Health and Well-Being of American Girls and Women" (report published by Women's Sports Foundation, East Meadow, NY, 2009), https://www.womenssportsfoundation.org/home/research/articles-and-reports/mental-and-physical-health/her-life-depends-on-it-ii.

3. https://www.womenssportsfoundation.org/home/research/articles-and-reports.

4. Kelly P. Troutman and Mikaela J. Dufur, "From High School Jocks to College Grads: Assessing the Long-Term Effects of High School Sport Participation on Females' Educational Attainment," *Youth Society* 38, no. 4 (June 2007): 443–62, http://yas.sagepub.com/content/38/4/443.abstract.

5. Jeffrey Thomas, "Equality in Sports Participation Benefits All, Says Expert," *IIP Digital*, April 17, 2008, http://iipdigital.usembassy.gov/st/english/article/2008/04/200804171153161cjsamoht0.6185572.html#axzz2x6Ivlq5N.

6. "Xavier Prep Sophomore Jessica Tonn Captures Second Straight 3200 Meter Title," AZ Track XC.com, May 9, 2008, http://az.milesplit.com/articles/18188#.Uy4NmL9D47A.

7. Jessica Tonn, interview by Kevin Selby at University of Washington Invitational, Seattle, January 27, 2013, http://www.flotrack.org/coverage/250018-2013-UW-Invitational/video/686290-Stanfords-Jessica-Tonn-hits-910-3k-PR-at-2013-UW-Invite#.Uy-v6xzr_qI.

8. Mary Healy Jonas, "Do Boys and Girls View Competition in Different Ways?" Melpomene Research Institute, 2013, http://www.footy4kids.co.uk/do-boys-and-girls-view-competition-in-different-ways.htm.

3. THE FAMILY THAT PLAYS TOGETHER STAYS TOGETHER

1. Jennifer A. Fredricks and Jacquelynne S. Eccles, "Parental Influences on Youth Involvement in Sports," in *Developmental Sport and Exercise Psychology: A Lifespan Perspective*, ed. Maureen R. Weiss (Morgantown, WV: Fitness Information Technology, 2004).

2. Gray, B. "Sports Help Dads, Daughters Bond, Study Says." March 13, 2014. *Health Day*. http://consumer.healthday.com/mental-health-information-25/behavior-health-news-56/sports-help-dads-daughters-bond-study-says-674142.html.

3. Gray, 2014.

4. Linda Nielsen, *Embracing Your Father: How to Build the Relationship You've Always Wanted with Your Dad* (New York: McGraw-Hill, 2004).

5. Pathways to the Podium Research Project, "Faster, Higher, Stronger . . . and Younger? Birth Order, Sibling Sport Participation, and Sport Expertise Development," *The Expert Advantage*, June 19, 2012, http://expertadvantage.wordpress.com/category/pathways-to-the-podium.

6. Pathways to the Podium Research Project, 2012.

7. Corinna Jenkins Tucker et al., "Association of Sibling Aggression with Child and Adolescent Mental Health," *Pediatrics* (2013), http://pediatrics.aappublications.org/content/early/2013/06/12/peds.2012-3801.

8. Anahad O'Connor, "When the Bully Is a Sibling," *New York Times*, June 17, 2013, http://well.blogs.nytimes.com/2013/06/17/when-the-bully-is-a-sibling.

9. Sam Bauman, "Sister Golfers Motivate Each Other and Team," *Northern Star*, April 16, 2013, http://northernstar.info/sports/columns/article_68726076-a6fa-11e2-83df-0019bb30f31a.html.

10. Associated Press, "Steven, Diana Lopez Earn Spot," ESPN, March 10, 2012, http://espn.go.com/olympics/story/_/id/7671208/steven-lopez-diana-lopez-earn-taekwondo-spots-london-mark-lopez-misses-cut.

4. ATHLETIC MOMS' CHALLENGES

1. Kelly O'Mara, "Can Women Come Back Faster after Pregnancy?" *Competitor*, October 3, 2013, http://running.competitor.com/2013/10/training/can-women-come-back-faster-after-pregnancy_61244.

2. Primary Research Assistant Kaisa Filppula, 2010, The Working Mother Report: What Moms Think: Career vs. Paycheck. www.workingmother.com/working-mother-research-institute

3. Petula Dvorak, "Olympic Moms Demonstrate How Women Can Have It All: Gold Medal, Cute Kids, Killer Abs," *Washington Post*, August 9, 2012, http://www.washingtonpost.com/local/us-olympic-moms-overcome-hurdles-and-have-the-killer-abs-and-medals-to-prove-it/2012/08/09/5c3c29f0-e223-11e1-a25e-15067bb31849_story.html.

4. Barbara Bronson Gray, "Sports Help Dads, Daughters Bond, Study Says," *HealthDay Reporter*, March 13, 2013, http://www.medicinenet.com/script/main/art.asp?articlekey=168491.

5. "Mom's Exercise during Pregnancy Gives Baby's Brain a Boost," CBC News, November 11, 2013, http://www.cbc.ca/news/health/mom-s-exercise-during-pregnancy-gives-baby-s-brain-a-boost-1.2422831.

6. "Kim Clijsters: Ready for the Mother of All Comebacks," *Independent*, August 5, 2009, http://www.independent.co.uk/sport/tennis/kim-clijsters-ready-for-the-mother-of-all-comebacks-1767285.html.

7. Louann Brizendine, *The Female Brain* (New York: Broadway Books, 2006), 95.

8. Denise Mann, "Pregnancy Brain: Myth or Reality?" WebMD, n.d., http://www.webmd.com/baby/features/memory_lapse_it_may_be_pregnancy_brain.

9. Kathleen Doheny, "'Mommy Brain' May Trigger Brain Growth," WebMD, n.d., http://www.webmd.com/baby/news/20101025/mommy-brain-may-trigger-brain-growth.

10. "Emma Garrard, Mom and Professional Triathlete Talks with GOTRIbal."

11. "Emma Garrard, Mom and Professional Triathlete Talks with GOTRIbal."

12. Danelle Kabush, Facebook post, 2013, https://www.facebook.com/groups/athletemoms.

13. Daniel G. Amen, *Unleash the Power of the Female Brain: Supercharging Yours for Better Health, Energy, Mood, Focus, and Sex* (New York: Harmony, 2013); Brizendine, *The Female Brain*.

5. ROMANTIC RELATIONSHIPS

1. Leslie Dobbins, "U.S. Women's Soccer Star Megan Rapinoe Talks Publicly about Girlfriend Sarah Walsh," *Shewired*, July 12, 2012, http://www.shewired.com/sports/2012/07/12/us-womens-soccer-star-megan-rapinoe-talks-publicly-about-girlfriend-sarah-walsh.

2. Trish Bendix, "Megan Rapinoe in *The New York Times,* Ryan Murphy Is Doing a Sex Show for HBO," *Afterellen*, April 11, 2013, http://www.afterellen.com/morning-brew-thurs-april-11-megan-rapinoe-in-the-new-york-times-ryan-murphy-is-doing-a-sex-show-for-hbo/04/2013.

3. Louann Brizendine, *The Female Brain* (New York: Broadway Books, 2006).

4. "Female Brain versus Male Brain," *NeuroRelay*, October 7, 2012, http://neurorelay.com/2012/10/07/female-brain-versus-male-brain.

6. BODY IMAGE OF FEMALE ATHLETES

1. Walter H. Kaye, MD, University of California, San Diego, School of Medicine, 2012 study, http://eatingdisorders.ucsd.edu/faculty/kaye.shtml.

2. "Dissatisfaction with Our Bodies and Eating Disorders" (online paper, University of Minnesota, Duluth, n.d.), http://www.d.umn.edu/~jvaleri/dissatisfaction%20with%20bodies.htm.

3. Joan Steidinger, PhD, "Perceptions of the Athletic Body," Disruptive Women in Health Care, July 27, 2012, http://www.disruptivewomen.net/2012/07/27/body-image-perceptions-of-the-athletic-body.

4. Caleb Daniloff, "Running on Empty," *Runner's World*, January 26, 2012, http://www.runnersworld.com/health/running-empty.

5. University of Michigan, "Disordered Eating and Eating Disorders," *Mitalk*, n.d., http://mitalk.umich.edu/article/11.

6. Walter Kaye and Danyale McCurdy, review of "Genetic Association of Recovery from Eating Disorders: The Role of GABA Receptor SNPs," by C. Bloss, W. Berrettini, A. Bergen, P. Magistretti, V. Duvvuri, M. Strober, H. Brandt, et al. *Neuropsychopharmacology*, 2011, http://eatingdisorders.ucsd.edu/research/genetics.

7. Daniloff, "Running on Empty."

8. "Walter H. Kaye, M.D.," University of California, San Diego, School of Medicine, http://eatingdisorders.ucsd.edu/faculty/kaye.shtml.

9. Hollie Avil, "London 2012 Olympics: Triathlete Hollie Avil Reveals Why She Has Decided to Bring an End to Her Promising Career," *Telegraph*, May 22,

2012, http://www.telegraph.co.uk/sport/olympics/triathlon/9280566/London-2012-Olympics-triathlete-Hollie-Avil-reveals-why-she-has-decided-to-bring-an-end-to-her-promising-career.html.

7. TEAM SPIRIT

1. Anni M., "Team Spirit!" Victoria Labalme, n.d., http://www.victorialabalme.com/communication_and_presentation_skills/?p=543.

2. Kathleen DeBoer, "A Balanced Attack," *Athletic Management*, February/March 2000, http://www.athleticmanagement.com/2007/03/19/a_balanced_attack/index.php.

3. Louann Brizendine, *The Female Brain* (New York: Broadway Books, 2006); Daniel G. Amen, *Unleash the Power of the Female Brain: Supercharging Yours for Better Health, Energy, Mood, Focus, and Sex* (New York: Harmony, 2013).

4. *Melpomene Journal* 11, no. 3 (Autumn 1992): 22.

5. Nicole M. LaVoi, "Girls Just Want to Have Fun, Too," *New York Times*, October 10, 2013, http://www.nytimes.com/roomfordebate/2013/10/10/childrens-sportslife-balance/girls-just-want-to-have-fun-too.

8. COACHES ARE CORNERSTONES

1. Stefanie Latham, "Coaching the Female Athlete," BBN Networks, February 23, 2012, http://www.slideshare.net/slatham0011/coaching-the-female-athlete.

2. Tony DiCicco, *Catch Them Being Good: Everything You Need to Know to Successfully Coach Girls* (New York: Penguin, 2002), 3.

3. Melina Timson-Katchis and Sophia Jowett, "The Athletic Triangle: Perceptions of Interpersonal Issues with Greek-Cypriot Coaches, Athletes, and Parents," Centro Esportivo Virtual, n.d., http://cev.org.br/biblioteca/the-athletic-triangle-perceptions-of-interpersonals-issues-with-greek-cypriot-coaches-athletes-and-parents.

4. "Parent, Coach, and Child: The Athletic Triangle," Women's Sports Foundation, n.d., https://www.womenssportsfoundation.org/en/home/athletes/for-athletes/know-your-rights/parent-resources/parent-coach-and-child-the-athletic-triangle.

9. PIONEERING FEMALE ATHLETES LAID THE FOUNDATION

1. Richard W. Riley and Norma V. Cantú, "Title IX, 25 Years of Progress" (report of the US Department of Education and Office for Civil Rights, June 1997), https://www2.ed.gov/pubs/TitleIX.

2. Sczcepanski, C. "Fewer men, more women riding?" September 3, 2013. The League of American Bicyclists Newsletter. http://bikeleague.org/content/fewer-men-more-women-riding.

3. Carolyn Szczepanski, "Fewer Men, More Women Riding?" League of American Bicyclists, September 3, 2013, http://bikeleague.org/content/fewer-men-more-women-riding.

4. Women's Sports Foundation, www.womenssportsfoundation.org.

5. "Jacquie Phelan: The Godmother of Women's Mountain Biking," *The Bicycle Story*, January 5, 2012, http://www.thebicyclestory.com/2012/01/jacquie-phelan-the-godmother-of-womens-mountain-biking/#more-353.

10. FEMALE COLLABORATIVE COMPETITION

1. See http://www.azlyrics.com/lyrics/drake/startedfromthebottom.html.

2. Mike Wise, "Tracy Barnes Makes Olympic Sacrifice for Her Sister Lanny," *Washington Post*, February 14, 2014, http://www.washingtonpost.com/sports/olympics/tracy-barnes-makes-olympic-sacrifice-for-her-sister-lanny/2014/02/14/5893d25a-95b2-11e3-9616-d367fa6ea99b_story.html.

3. See https://www.facebook.com/groups/athletemoms.

BIBLIOGRAPHY

Amen, Daniel G. *Unleash the Power of the Female Brain: Supercharging Yours for Better Health, Energy, Mood, Focus, and Sex.* New York: Harmony, 2013.

Associated Press. "Steven, Diana Lopez Earn Spot." ESPN. March 10, 2012. http://espn.go.com/olympics/story/_/id/7671208/steven-lopez-diana-lopez-earn-taekwondo-spots-london-mark-lopez-misses-cut.

Avil, Hollie. "London 2012 Olympics: Triathlete Hollie Avil Reveals Why She Has Decided to Bring an End to Her Promising Career." *Telegraph.* May 22, 2012. http://www.telegraph.co.uk/sport/olympics/triathlon/9280566/London-2012-Olympics-triathlete-Hollie-Avil-reveals-why-she-has-decided-to-bring-an-end-to-her-promising-career.html.

Bauman, Sam. "Sister Golfers Motivate Each Other and Team." *Northern Star.* April 16, 2013. http://northernstar.info/sports/columns/article_68726076-a6fa-11e2-83df-0019bb30f31a.html.

Bendix, Trish. "Megan Rapinoe in *The New York Times,* Ryan Murphy Is Doing a Sex Show for HBO." *Afterellen.* April 11, 2013. http://www.afterellen.com/morning-brew-thurs-april-11-megan-rapinoe-in-the-new-york-times-ryan-murphy-is-doing-a-sex-show-for-hbo/04/2013.

Brizendine, Louann. *The Female Brain.* New York: Broadway Books, 2006.

Cloud, John. "Why Girls Have BFFs and Boys Hang Out in Packs." *Time.* July 17, 2009. http://content.time.com/time/health/article/0,8599,1911103,00.html.

Cook, Gareth. "The Secret Language Code." *Scientific American.* August 16, 2011. http://www.scientificamerican.com/article/the-secret-language-code.

Daniloff, Caleb. "Running on Empty." *Runner's World.* January 26, 2012. http://www.runnersworld.com/health/running-empty.

DeBoer, Kathleen. "A Balanced Attack." *Athletic Management.* February/March 2000. http://www.athleticmanagement.com/2007/03/19/a_balanced_attack/index.php.

DiCicco, Tony. *Catch Them Being Good: Everything You Need to Know to Successfully Coach Girls.* New York: Penguin, 2002.

"Dissatisfaction with Our Bodies and Eating Disorders." Online paper, University of Minnesota, Duluth, n.d., http://www.d.umn.edu/~jvaleri/dissatisfaction%20with%20bodies.htm.

Dobbins, Leslie. "U.S. Women's Soccer Star Megan Rapinoe Talks Publicly about Girlfriend Sarah Walsh." *Shewired.* July 12, 2012. http://www.shewired.com/sports/2012/07/12/us-womens-soccer-star-megan-rapinoe-talks-publicly-about-girlfriend-sarah-walsh.

Doheny, Kathleen. "'Mommy Brain' May Trigger Brain Growth." WebMD. N.d. http://www.webmd.com/baby/news/20101025/mommy-brain-may-trigger-brain-growth.

Dvorak, Petula. "Olympic Moms Demonstrate How Women Can Have It All: Gold Medal, Cute Kids, Killer Abs." *Washington Post.* August 9, 2012. http://www.washingtonpost.com/

local/us-olympic-moms-overcome-hurdles-and-have-the-killer-abs-and-medals-to-prove-it/
2012/08/09/5c3c29f0-e223-11e1-a25e-15067bb31849_story.html.

"Emma Garrard, Mom and Professional Triathlete Talks with GOTRIbal." GOTRIbal. November 11, 2013. http://www.gotribalnow.com/blog/emma-garrard-mom-and-professional-triathlete-talks-gotribal.

"Female Brain versus Male Brain." *NeuroRelay*. October 7, 2012. http://neurorelay.com/2012/10/07/female-brain-versus-male-brain.

Fitzpatrick, Deirdre. "Team USA Sisters Compete in Olympic Swimming." WXII12.com. August 7, 2012. http://www.wxii12.com/sports/2014-olympics/Team-USA-sisters-compete-in-Olympic-swimming/16005138.

Fredricks, Jennifer A., and Jacquelynne S. Eccles. "Parental Influences on Youth Involvement in Sports." In *Developmental Sport and Exercise Psychology: A Lifespan Perspective*, edited by Maureen R. Weiss. Morgantown, WV: Fitness Information Technology, 2004.

"How Male and Female Brains Differ." WebMD. N.d. http://www.webmd.com/balance/features/how-male-female-brains-differ.

"Jacquie Phelan: The Godmother of Women's Mountain Biking." *The Bicycle Story*. January 5, 2012. http://www.thebicyclestory.com/2012/01/jacquie-phelan-the-godmother-of-womens-mountain-biking/#more-353.

Jonas, Mary Healy. "Do Boys and Girls View Competition in Different Ways?" Melpomene Research Institute. 2013. http://www.footy4kids.co.uk/do-boys-and-girls-view-competition-in-different-ways.htm.

Jordan, Judith V., Alexandra G. Kaplan, Jean Baker Miller, Irene P. Stiver, and Janet L. Surrey. *Women's Growth in Connection: Writings from the Stone Center*. Boston: Guilford Press, 1991.

Kaye, Walter, and Danyale McCurdy. Review of "Genetic Association of Recovery from Eating Disorders: The Role of GABA Receptor SNPs," by C. Bloss, W. Berrettini, A. Bergen, P. Magistretti, V. Duvvuri, M. Strober, H. Brandt, et al., *Neuropsychopharmacology* (2011). http://eatingdisorders.ucsd.edu/research/genetics.

Latham, Stefanie. "Coaching the Female Athlete." BBN Networks. February 23, 2012. http://www.slideshare.net/slatham0011/coaching-the-female-athlete.

LaVoi, Nicole M. "Girls Just Want to Have Fun, Too." *New York Times*. October 10, 2013. http://www.nytimes.com/roomfordebate/2013/10/10/childrens-sportslife-balance/girls-just-want-to-have-fun-too.

M., Anni. "Team Spirit!" Victoria Labalme. N.d. http://www.victorialabalme.com/communication_and_presentation_skills/?p=543.

Mann, Denise. "Pregnancy Brain: Myth or Reality?" WebMD. N.d. http://www.webmd.com/baby/features/memory_lapse_it_may_be_pregnancy_brain.

"Mom's Exercise during Pregnancy Gives Baby's Brain a Boost." CBC News. November 11, 2013. http://www.cbc.ca/news/health/mom-s-exercise-during-pregnancy-gives-baby-s-brain-a-boost-1.2422831.

Nielsen, Linda. *Embracing Your Father: How to Build the Relationship You've Always Wanted with Your Dad*. New York: McGraw-Hill, 2004.

O'Connor, Anahad. "When the Bully Is a Sibling." *New York Times*. June 17, 2013. http://well.blogs.nytimes.com/2013/06/17/when-the-bully-is-a-sibling.

O'Mara, Kelly. "Can Women Come Back Faster after Pregnancy?" *Competitor*. October 3, 2013. http://running.competitor.com/2013/10/training/can-women-come-back-faster-after-pregnancy_61244.

"Parent, Coach, and Child: The Athletic Triangle." Women's Sports Foundation. N.d. https://www.womenssportsfoundation.org/en/home/athletes/for-athletes/know-your-rights/parent-resources/parent-coach-and-child-the-athletic-triangle.

Pathways to the Podium Research Project. "Faster, Higher, Stronger . . . and Younger? Birth Order, Sibling Sport Participation, and Sport Expertise Development." *The Expert Advantage*. June 19, 2012. http://expertadvantage.wordpress.com/category/pathways-to-the-podium.

Polivy, Jane, and C. Peter Herman. "Causes of Eating Disorders." *Annual Review of Psychology* 53 (2002): 187–213.

"The Real 'Mommy Brain': New Mothers Grew Bigger Brains within Months of Giving Birth." American Psychological Association. October 20, 2010. http://www.apa.org/news/press/releases/2010/10/mommy-brain.aspx.

Riley, Richard W., and Norma V. Cantú. "Title IX, 25 Years of Progress." Report of the US Department of Education and Office for Civil Rights, June 1997. https://www2.ed.gov/pubs/TitleIX.

Sax, Leonard. Why Gender Matters: What Parents and Teachers Need to Know about the Emerging Science of Sex Differences. New York: Doubleday, 2005.

Staurowsky, J. E., M. J. DeSousa, G. Ducher, N. Gentner, K. E. Miller, S. Shakib, N. Theberge, and N. Williams. "Her Life Depends on It II: Sport, Physical Activity, and the Health and Well-Being of American Girls and Women." Report published by Women's Sports Foundation, East Meadow, NY, 2009. https://www.womenssportsfoundation.org/home/research/articles-and-reports/mental-and-physical-health/her-life-depends-on-it-ii.

Szczepanski, Carolyn. "Fewer Men, More Women Riding?" League of American Bicyclists. September 3, 2013. http://bikeleague.org/content/fewer-men-more-women-riding.

Tannen, Deborah. You Just Don't Understand: Women and Men in Conversation. New York: William Morrow and Company, 1990.

Taylor, Shelley E. The Tending Instinct: Women, Men, and the Biology of Relationships. New York: Henry Holt and Company, 2002.

Taylor, Shelley E., Laura Cousino Klein, Brian P. Lewis, Tara L. Gruenewald, Regan A. R. Gurung, and John A. Updegraff. "Biobehavioral Responses to Stress in Females: Tend-and-Befriend, Not Fight-or-Flight." Psychological Review 107, no. 3 (2000): 411–29. http://taylorlab.psych.ucla.edu/2000_Biobehavioral%20responses%20to%20stress%20in%20females_tend-and-befriend.pdf.

Thomas, Jeffrey. "Equality in Sports Participation Benefits All, Says Expert." IIP Digital. April 17, 2008. http://iipdigital.usembassy.gov/st/english/article/2008/04/200804171153161cjsamoht0.6185572.html#axzz2x6Ivlq5N.

Timson-Katchis, Melina, and Sophia Jowett. "The Athletic Triangle: Perceptions of Interpersonal Issues with Greek-Cypriot Coaches, Athletes, and Parents." Centro Esportivo Virtual. N.d. http://cev.org.br/biblioteca/the-athletic-triangle-perceptions-of-interpersonals-issues-with-greek-cypriot-coaches-athletes-and-parents.

Tonn, Jessica. Interview by Kevin Selby at University of Washington Invitational, Seattle. January 27, 2013. http://www.flotrack.org/coverage/250018-2013-UW-Invitational/video/686290-Stanfords-Jessica-Tonn-hits-910-3k-PR-at-2013-UW-Invite#.Uy-v6xzr_qI.

Troutman, Kelly P., and Mikaela J. Dufur. "From High School Jocks to College Grads: Assessing the Long-Term Effects of High School Sport Participation on Females' Educational Attainment." Youth Society 38, no. 4 (June 2007): 443–62. http://yas.sagepub.com/content/38/4/443.abstract.

Tucker, Corinna Jenkins, David Finkelhor, Heather Turner, and Anne Shattuck. "Association of Sibling Aggression with Child and Adolescent Mental Health." Pediatrics (2013). http://pediatrics.aappublications.org/content/early/2013/06/12/peds.2012-3801.

University of Michigan. "Disordered Eating and Eating Disorders." Mitalk. N.d. http://mitalk.umich.edu/article/11.

Wilson Sporting Goods Co. "The Wilson Report: Moms, Dads, Daughters, and Sports." Report presented by Wilson Sporting Goods Co. and Women's Sports Foundation. 1998. https://www.womenssportsfoundation.org/en/home/research/articles-and-reports/mental-and-physical-health/moms-dads-daughters-and-sports.

Wise, Mike. "Tracy Barnes Makes Olympic Sacrifice for her Sister Lanny." Washington Post. February 14, 2014. http://www.washingtonpost.com/sports/olympics/tracy-barnes-makes-olympic-sacrifice-for-her-sister-lanny/2014/02/14/5893d25a-95b2-11e3-9616-d367fa6ea99b_story.html.

Wyshynski, Greg. "Kerri Walsh Jennings and Misty May-Treanor on Their 'Marriage Counseling.'" Yahoo! Sports. July 30, 2012. https://sports.yahoo.com/blogs/fourth-place-medal/kerri-walsh-jennings-misty-may-treanor-marriage-counseling-002204382--oly.html.

"Xavier Prep Sophomore Jessica Tonn Captures Second Straight 3200 Meter Title." AZ Track XC.com. May 9, 2008. http://az.milesplit.com/articles/18188#.Uy4NmL9D47A.

INDEX

AASP. *See* Association of Applied Sports Psychology

absent and removed type, of mothers, 45

academic achievement, 22

actively supportive relationship model, 81–82

adjourning stage of team dynamics, 114–115

advocacy. *See* pioneering women athletes

aggression, 10, 15, 33, 52, 75

aggressive and pressuring type, of mothers, 44–45

Allred, Alex, 58

Amen, Daniel, 16, 158; on competition, 32

amenorrhea, 102

analytical and supportive type, of mothers, 43

Anderson, Alyssa, 51

Anderson, Haley, 51

anorexia athletica, 99

anorexia nervosa, 97–99

Association of Applied Sports Psychology (AASP), 136; Conference 2012, 17

athletic couples, 71; actively supportive, 81–82; brain comparisons and, 74–77; dynamics, 77–78; introduced to sport by partner, 82; mental strategies for, 85; mutually supportive in different sports, 84; mutually supportive in same sport, 79–80; quietly supportive, 83; supportive, 73–74; types, 78–84

athletic moms, 42, 43, 57–58; committed strong, 66–67; emotions and, 64; evolution of, 67–69; guilt and, 64; mental skills after pregnancy, 65–66; mental strategies for, 69–70; mind of, 61–65; in 1980s, 67–68; in 1990s, 68–69; partners of, 64; physical challenges, 59–61. *See also* pregnancy

athletic triangle, 134–136

Avil, Hollie, 98

Bagley, Shana, 92

Barnes, Lanny, 158–159

Barnes, Tracy, 158–159

Bassman, Andrea, 12

Bayles, Charlene, 67–68

befriend, 11. *See also* tend-and-befriend

best friends, 27; benefits of, 24–27; BFFs versus buddies in arms, 29–31; competition and, 24; lasting, 24–27; mental strategies for, 34–35; teenage girls and, 19–20, 20–24

Biefeld, Joy, 148

biology, teenage, 33

body image, 87–88, 104; basics of, 88–90; eating and, 92–93; fitness and, 90–92; mental strategies for, 104–105; mothers and, 88; Olympic Games 2012 and, 87, 93. *See also* disordered eating; eating disorders

Body Positive, 90

CONTRIBUTORS

Thank you to all these wonderful interviewees!

DIRECT CONTRIBUTORS

Shana Bagley—sailing, strongman
Charlene Bayles—runner
Claudia Bouvier—pro big-mountain skiing
Ana Braga-Levaggi—ultrarunner
Karen Brems—Olympic cyclist
Rosie Casals—pro tennis
Martha Cederstrom—former elite and pioneering ultrarunner
Avigiel Cohen—Cal Berkeley women's basketball
Maili Costa—runner
Katheryn Curi Mattis—pro cyclist
Donna de Varona—Olympic gold medalist swimmer and first president/chairman of the Women's Sport's Foundation
Alison Dunlap—Olympic road and mountain biker, pro mountain biker
Honor Fetherston—national Masters road runner
Rebecca Fong—high school softball
Samantha Gash—Australian pro ultrarunner
Lindsay Gottlieb—Cal Berkeley women's basketball head coach
Ken Grace—community college track-and-field coach

Gina Grain—Canadian Olympic cyclist, pro cyclist

Georgia Gould—Olympic 2012 bronze medalist

Sofia Hamilton—junior national mountain biker

Makena Hayden—high school volleyball player

C. J. Healy—head and assistant head basketball coach

Barbra Higgins—Panamanian Olympic fencer

Caren Horstmeyer—former Santa Clara University and Cal Berkeley women's basketball head coach

Jeri Howland—elite triathlete

Luca Jampolsky—first female Stanford gymnast

Lorraine Jarvis—elite track cyclist

Stacey Johnson—Olympic fencer

Kim Juarez—runner

Danelle Kabush—Canadian pro XTERRA triathlete

Dr. Haleh Kashani—director of eating disorders program

Kristine Lilly—Olympic and pro soccer player, member of "Fab Five"

Lisa Lopez—all-American miler and former captain of Cal Berkeley cross-country

Mikayla Lyles—Cal Berkeley women's basketball

Julia Mancuso—Olympic gold, double silver, bronze medalist, pro skier

Erin Maxwell—pro sailing (4.7 meter boats)

Tracy McCullough—tennis

Mary McLain—tennis

Ann Meyers Drysdale—Olympic silver medalist and pro basketball

Meredith Miller—pro road cyclist

Carole Oglesby—1950s softball player and grandmother of sports psychology

Jennifer Pharr Davis—holder of overall record through-hiker of Appalachian Trail

Aria Pogni—high school softball

Jamie Rivers—elite trail runner

Kami Semick—pro ultrarunner

Mackinzie Stanley—high school and team mountain biker and runner

Jennifer Steinman—film director

Marla Streb—pro downhill mountain biker

Lisa Tamati—Kiwi pro ultrarunner

Christine Thorburn—Olympic and pro road cyclist

Julia Violich—elite mountain biker and coach
Kristin Wentzel—junior world championship 8+ rower
Kathy Winkler—elite Masters triathlete
Mike Woitalia—soccer journalist and youth coach

INDIRECT CONTRIBUTORS

Gabrielle Anderson—Swiss Olympic runner
Rick Bobington—Paralympic coach
Lisa Bouvier—equestrian
Irene D'Agostino—eighty-eight-year-old competitive swimmer
Kristin Drumm—elite road cyclist
Pam Fernandez—Paralympic coach
Gena Harper—aspiring Paralympic athlete
Eva Hayden—alpine skier
Rachel Lloyd—elite runner and mountain biker
Shelley Olds—Olympic and European pro road cyclist
Eve Pell—elite runner
Juliana Rende—showcasing snowboarder
Tyler Stewart—pro triathlete
Christine Waldron—runner